Pulmonary Embolism in the ICU

Editors

BHARAT AWSARE
MICHAEL BARAM
GENO MERLI

CRITICAL CARE CLINICS

www.criticalcare.theclinics.com

Consulting Editor
JOHN A. KELLUM

July 2020 • Volume 36 • Number 3

ELSEVIER

1600 John F. Kennedy Boulevard • Suite 1800 • Philadelphia, Pennsylvania, 19103-2899

http://www.theclinics.com

CRITICAL CARE CLINICS Volume 36, Number 3
July 2020 ISSN 0749-0704, ISBN-13: 978-0-323-71293-4

Editor: Kerry Holland
Developmental Editor: Casey Potter

Critical Care Clinics (ISSN: 0749-0704) is published quarterly by Elsevier Inc., 360 Park Avenue South, New York, NY 10010-1710. Months of issue are January, April, July, and October. Business and Editorial Offices: 1600 John F. Kennedy Blvd., Suite 1800, Philadelphia, PA 19103-2899. Customer Service Office: 6277 Sea Harbor Drive, Orlando, FL 32887-4800. Periodicals postage paid at New York, NY and additional mailing offices. Subscription prices are $250.00 per year for US individuals, $683.00 per year for US institutions, $100.00 per year for US students and residents, $285.00 per year for Canadian individuals, $856.00 per year for Canadian institutions, $318.00 per year for international individuals, $856.00 per year for international institutions, $100.00 per year for Canadian students/residents, and $150.00 per year for foreign students/residents. To receive student/resident rate, orders must be accompanied by name of affiliated institution, date of term, and the signature of program/residency coordinator on institution letterhead. Orders will be billed at individual rate until proof of status is received. Foreign air speed delivery is included in all *Clinics* subscription prices. All prices are subject to change without notice. POSTMASTER: Send address changes to *Critical Care Clinics*, Elsevier Periodicals Customer Service, 11830 Westline Industrial Drive, St. Louis, MO 63146. **Customer Service: 1-800-654-2452 (US). From outside of the US, call 1-314-447-8871. Fax: 1-314-447-8029. E-mail: journalscustomerservice-usa@elsevier.com (for print support) or journalsonlinesupport-usa@elsevier.com (for online support).**

Reprints. For copies of 100 or more of articles in this publication, please contact the Commercial Reprints Department, Elsevier Inc., 360 Park Avenue South, New York, NY 10010-1710. Tel.: 212-633-3874; Fax: 212-633-3820; E-mail: reprints@elsevier.com.

Critical Care Clinics is also published in Spanish by Editorial Inter-Medica, Junin 917, 1er A, 1113, Buenos Aires, Argentina.

Critical Care Clinics is covered in *MEDLINE/PubMed (Index Medicus)*, *EMBASE/Excerpta Medica*, *Current Concepts/Clinical Medicine*, *ISI/BIOMED*, and *Chemical Abstracts*.

Contributors

CONSULTING EDITOR

JOHN A. KELLUM, MD, MCCM
Professor, Critical Care Medicine, Medicine, Bioengineering and Clinical and Translational Science, Director, Center for Critical Care Nephrology, The Clinical Research Investigation and Systems Modeling of Acute Illness (CRISMA) Center, Vice Chair for Research, Department of Critical Care Medicine, University of Pittsburgh School of Medicine, Pittsburgh, Pennsylvania, USA

EDITORS

BHARAT AWSARE, MD
Director of Medical Intensive Care Unit, Director, Thomas Jefferson Pulmonary Embolism Response Team, Clinical Associate Professor of Medicine, Department of Medicine, Division of Pulmonary and Critical Care, Jefferson University Hospital, Korman Lung Institute, Philadelphia, Pennsylvania, USA

MICHAEL BARAM, MD
Associate Fellowship Director for Pulmonary and Critical Care Training, Associate Professor, Department of Medicine, Division of Pulmonary and Critical Care, Jefferson University Hospital, Korman Lung Institute, Philadelphia, Pennsylvania, USA

GENO MERLI, MD
Senior Vice President and Associate Chief Medical Officer, Professor of Medicine, Department of Medicine and Surgery, Division of Vascular Medicine, Jefferson University Hospital, Philadelphia, Pennsylvania, USA

AUTHORS

BHARAT AWSARE, MD
Director of Medical Intensive Care Unit, Director, Thomas Jefferson Pulmonary Embolism Response Team, Clinical Associate Professor of Medicine, Department of Medicine, Division of Pulmonary and Critical Care, Jefferson University Hospital, Korman Lung Institute, Philadelphia, Pennsylvania, USA

MICHAEL BARAM, MD
Associate Fellowship Director for Pulmonary and Critical Care Training, Associate Professor, Department of Medicine, Division of Pulmonary and Critical Care, Jefferson University Hospital, Korman Lung Institute, Philadelphia, Pennsylvania, USA

JOHN R. BARTHOLOMEW, MD, MSVM, FACC
Professor of Medicine, Cleveland Clinic Lerner College of Medicine, Section Head, Vascular Medicine, Department of Cardiovascular Medicine, Cleveland Clinic, Cleveland, Ohio, USA

VANESSA M. BAZAN, BSc
College of Medicine, University of Kentucky, Lexington, Kentucky, USA

RICHARD N. CHANNICK, MD
Co-Director, Pulmonary Vascular Disease Program, Director, Acute and Chronic Thromboembolic Disease Program, Division of Pulmonary and Critical Care, University of California, Los Angeles, David Geffen School of Medicine, Los Angeles, California, USA

DALE SHELTON DEAS, MD
Integrated Resident, Cardiothoracic Surgery, Division of Cardiothoracic Surgery, Emory University, Atlanta, Georgia, USA

JAMES DOUKETIS, MD, FRCPC
Department of Medicine, St. Joseph's Healthcare Hamilton, McMaster University, Hamilton, Ontario, Canada

OREN FRIEDMAN, MD
Associate Professor of Medicine, Cedars-Sinai Medical Center, Los Angeles, California, USA

SHANNON GARVEY, MS
Boston University School of Medicine, Boston, Massachusetts, USA

SONIA JASUJA, MD
Division of Pulmonary and Critical Care, University of California, Los Angeles, David Geffen School of Medicine, Los Angeles, California, USA

CHRISTOPHER KABRHEL, MD, MPH
Director, Center for Vascular Emergencies, Department of Emergency Medicine, Massachusetts General Hospital, MGH Endowed Chair in Emergency Medicine, Professor of Emergency Medicine, Harvard Medical School, Boston, Massachusetts, USA

ERIC KAPLOVITCH, MD, FRCPC
Department of Medicine, University Health Network and Sinai Health System, University of Toronto, Toronto, Ontario, Canada

BRENT KEELING, MD, FACS, FACC
Associate Professor of Surgery, Division of Cardiothoracic Surgery, Emory University, Atlanta, Georgia, USA

GENO MERLI, MD
Senior Vice President and Associate Chief Medical Officer, Professor of Medicine, Department of Medicine and Surgery, Division of Vascular Medicine, Jefferson University Hospital, Philadelphia, Pennsylvania, USA

SEBASTIEN MIRANDA, MD
University of Ottawa, Ontario, Canada; Department of Internal Medicine, Vascular and Thrombosis Unit, Rouen University Hospital, Normandie University, UNIROUEN, INSERM U1096, Rouen, France

THOMAS MOUMNEH, MD
Department of Emergency Medicine, University Hospital of Angers, MITOVASC Institute, UMR CNRS 6015 UMR INSERM 1083, Angers University, Angers, France; University of Ottawa, Ontario, Canada

PETER RODGERS-FISCHL, MD
Thoracic Surgery I-6 Residency Program, PGY4, Division of Cardiothoracic Surgery, Kentucky Clinic, UK Health Care, Lexington, Kentucky, USA

RACHEL ROSOVSKY, MD, MPH
Division of Hematology, Department of Medicine, Massachusetts General Hospital, Assistant Professor of Medicine, Harvard Medical School, Boston, Massachusetts, USA

DAVID M. RUOHONIEMI, BS
Department of Radiology, Division of Interventional Radiology, NYU Grossman School of Medicine, New York, New York, USA

JOSEPH R. SHAW, MD
Ottawa Blood Disease Centre, The Ottawa Hospital, Ottawa, Canada

AKHILESH K. SISTA, MD
Department of Radiology, Division of Interventional Radiology, NYU Grossman School of Medicine, New York, New York, USA

VICTOR F. TAPSON, MD
Professor of Medicine, Associate Director, Pulmonary and Critical Care Medicine, Cedars-Sinai Medical Center, Los Angeles, California, USA

AARON S. WEINBERG, MD, MPhil
Assistant Professor of Medicine, Cedars-Sinai Medical Center, Los Angeles, California, USA

PHILIP S. WELLS, MD, FRCP(C), MSc
Chief/Chair, Department of Medicine, University of Ottawa, Ottawa Hospital Research Institute, Ottawa, Ontario, Canada

STEVEN ZHAO, MD
Division of Pulmonary and Critical Care Medicine, Cedars-Sinai Medical Center, Los Angeles, California, USA

JOSEPH B. ZWISCHENBERGER, MD
Chair Emeritus, Department of Surgery, University of Kentucky, University of Kentucky Medical Center, Lexington, Kentucky, USA

Contents

Erratum xi

Preface: Intensive Care Units as a Place to Manage Pulmonary Emboli xiii

Bharat Awsare, Michael Baram, and Geno Merli

Pulmonary Embolism in Intensive Care Unit 427

Michael Baram, Bharat Awsare, and Geno Merli

Management of pulmonary embolism (PE) has become more complex due to the expanded role of catheter-based therapies, surgical thrombectomies, and cardiac assist technologies, such as right ventricular assist devices and extracorporeal support. Due to the heterogeneity of PE, a multidisciplinary team approach is necessary. The manifestation of PE response teams are in response to this complex need and similar to the proliferation of stroke, trauma, and rapid response teams. Intensive care units are an ideal location for formulating a comprehensive treatment plan that necessitates an interaction between multiple specialties. This article addresses the unique needs of critically ill patients with PE.

Risk Stratification of Pulmonary Embolism 437

Thomas Moumneh, Philip S. Wells, and Sebastien Miranda

Given the broad treatment options, risk stratification of pulmonary embolism is a highly desirable component of management. The ideal tool identifies patients at risk of death from the original or recurrent pulmonary embolism. Using all-cause death in the first 30-days after pulmonary embolism diagnosis as a surrogate, clinical parameters, biomarkers, and radiologic evidence of right ventricular dysfunction and strain are predictive. However, no study has demonstrated improved mortality rates after implementation of a risk stratification strategy to guide treatment. Further research should use better methodology to study prognosis and test new management strategies in patients at high risk for death.

Overview of Management of Intermediate- and High-Risk Pulmonary Embolism 449

Victor F. Tapson and Aaron S. Weinberg

Anticoagulation is the cornerstone of acute pulmonary embolism (PE) therapy. Intermediate-risk (submassive) or high-risk (massive) PE patients have higher mortality than low-risk patients. It is generally accepted that high-risk PE patients should be considered for more aggressive therapy. Intermediate-risk patients can be subdivided, although more than simply categorizing the patient is required to guide therapy. Therapeutic approaches depend on a prompt, detailed evaluation, and PE response teams may help with rapid assessment and initiation of therapy. More clinical trial data are needed to guide clinicians in the management of acute intermediate- and high-risk PE patients.

Thrombolysis in Pulmonary Embolism: An Evidence-Based Approach to Treating Life-Threatening Pulmonary Emboli 465

Eric Kaplovitch, Joseph R. Shaw, and James Douketis

Acute pulmonary embolism (PE) is associated with high in-hospital morbidity and mortality, both via cardiorespiratory decompensation and the bleeding complications of treatment. Thrombolytic therapy can be life-saving in those with high-risk PE, but requires careful patient selection. Patients with PE and systemic arterial hypotension ("massive PE") should receive thrombolytic therapy unless severe contraindications are present. Patients with PE and right ventricular dysfunction/injury, but without hypotension ("submassive PE"), should be considered for thrombolysis on a case-by-case basis, considering bleeding risk, cardiac biomarkers, echocardiography, and most importantly, clinical status.

Interventional Radiology Therapy: Inferior Vena Cava Filter and Catheter-based Therapies 481

David M. Ruohoniemi and Akhilesh K. Sista

Endovascular management of pulmonary embolism can be divided into therapeutic and prophylactic treatments. Prophylactic treatment includes inferior vena cava filter placement, whereas endovascular therapeutic interventions include an array of catheter-directed therapies. The indications for both modalities have evolved over the last decade as new evidence has become available.

Surgical Pulmonary Embolectomy 497

Dale Shelton Deas and Brent Keeling

Surgical pulmonary embolectomy has a storied history in the domain of cardiothoracic surgery. This article provides insight on the history, current data, and future directions of surgical pulmonary embolectomy.

Management of Right Ventricular Failure in Pulmonary Embolism 505

Steven Zhao and Oren Friedman

Acute right ventricular failure remains the leading cause of mortality associated with acute pulmonary embolism (PE). This article reviews the pathophysiology behind acute right ventricular failure and strategies for managing right ventricular failure in acute PE. Immediate clot reduction via systemic thrombolytics, catheter based procedures, or surgery is always advocated for unstable patients. While waiting to mobilize these resources, it often becomes necessary to support the RV with vasoactive medications. Clinicians should carefully assess volume status and use caution with volume resuscitation. Right ventricular assist devices may have an expanding role in the future.

Supportive Therapy: Extracorporeal Membrane Oxygenation   517

Vanessa M. Bazan, Peter Rodgers-Fischl, and Joseph B. Zwischenberger

Acute high-risk pulmonary embolism (PE) is characterized by life-threatening hemodynamic instability that may lead to refractory cardiac arrest. Recently, extracorporeal membrane oxygenation (ECMO) has been used to provide primary cardiopulmonary support for select high-risk PE patients or before surgical embolectomy. This article reviews the growing body of literature regarding ECMO support of acute high-risk PE.

Special Considerations in Pulmonary Embolism: Clot-in-Transit and Incidental
Pulmonary Embolism   531

Christopher Kabrhel, Rachel Rosovsky, and Shannon Garvey

This article describes 2 relatively rare, but complex situations in pulmonary embolism (PE): clot-in-transit (CIT), incidental PE (IPE). CIT describes a venous thromboembolism that has become lodged in the right heart. CIT is associated with high mortality and presents unique challenges in management. Incidental PE (IPE) describes PE diagnosed on imaging performed for another indication. The treatment is complex because there is often a disconnect between the PE severity on imaging and lack of severity of the clinical presentation. We summarize the available literature and aid clinicians as they manage patients with PE across the clinical severity spectrum.

Pulmonary Embolism in the Intensive Care Unit: Therapy in Subpopulations   547

John R. Bartholomew

The optimal management of a submassive or massive pulmonary embolism (PE) during pregnancy is unclear because of a lack of large clinical trials. Evaluation of the patient who may be a candidate for more aggressive therapy includes the use of biomarkers and echocardiogram for risk stratification. PE Response teams (PERTs) have gained increasing acceptance by the medical community and are being implemented in hospitals in the United States and worldwide. PERTs bring together a team of specialists from different disciplines to enhance decision-making in the patient with acute submassive and massive PE.

Post-Intensive Care Unit Follow-up of Pulmonary Embolism   561

Sonia Jasuja and Richard N. Channick

The post-intensive care unit follow-up of patients hospitalized with pulmonary embolism is crucial to the comprehensive care of these patients. This article discusses the recommended duration of intensive care unit stay after high-intermediate risk or high-risk pulmonary embolism, duration of anticoagulation after venous thromboembolism event, retrieval of inferior vena cava filters, post-hospitalization follow-up and assessment of right ventricular function, and assessment for chronic thromboembolic pulmonary hypertension, chronic thromboembolic disease, and post–pulmonary embolism syndrome.

CRITICAL CARE CLINICS

FORTHCOMING ISSUES

October 2020
Part I: Enhanced Recovery in the ICU After Cardiac Surgery
Part II: New Developments in Cardiopulmonary Resuscitation
Daniel Engelman and Clif Callaway, *Editors*

January 2021
Part I: Critical Care of the Cancer Patient
Part II: Geriatric Critical Care
Stephen M. Pastores and Wendy R. Greene, *Editors*

April 2021
Acute Kidney Injury
John A. Kellum and Dana Furham, *Editors*

RECENT ISSUES

April 2020
Coagulation/Endothelial Dysfunction
Hernando Gomez Danies and Joseph A. Carcillo, *Editors*

January 2020
Biomarkers in Critical Care
Mitchell M. Levy, *Editor*

October 2019
Intensive Care Unit in Disaster
Marie Baldisseri, Mary J. Reed, and Randy Wax, *Editors*

THE CLINICS ARE AVAILABLE ONLINE!
Access your subscription at:
www.theclinics.com

Erratum

Please note the following correction in the article Opal SM, Wittebole X. Biomarkers of Infection and Sepsis. Crit Care Clin 2020;36(1):11-22: Reference number 65 should be Miller RR, Lopansri BK, Burke JP, et al. Validation of a host response assay, SeptiCyte LAB, for discriminating sepsis from systemic inflammatory syndrome in the ICU. Am J Respir Crit Care Med 2018;198(7):904-13.

https://doi.org/10.1016/j.ccc.2020.05.001

Preface

Intensive Care Units as a Place to Manage Pulmonary Emboli

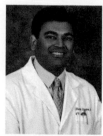   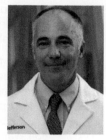   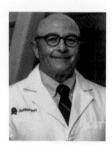

Bharat Awsare, MD   Michael Baram, MD   Geno Merli, MD

Editors

There was once a time when the main considerations for the acute treatment of pulmonary emboli (PE) were anticoagulation, inferior vena caval interruption, and thrombolytics. The diagnosis, risk-stratification, treatment, and follow-up of PE has become more complicated. Due to the heterogeneity of PE patients (medical, oncology, orthopedics, surgery, neurosurgery, pediatrics, and obstetrics), a variety of alternate options began to develop. The management of PE became more complex due to the expanded role of catheter-based therapies, surgical thrombectomies, and cardiac-assist technologies, such as right ventricular-assist devices and extracorporeal support. Formulating a comprehensive treatment plan now necessitates an interaction between multiple specialties and departments. The intensive care unit (ICU) is designed not only to provide support for the most critically ill but also to facilitate the multidisciplinary care provided by intensivists, hematologists, vascular specialists, cardiologists, interventional radiologists, pharmacists, and cardiothoracic surgeons. When an institution engages the multiple disciplines with PE expertise to develop algorithms of best practice and processes of care, patient care can be improved through optimized management of local resources. The same organized team can develop institutional algorithms as well as provide direct patient care. The most complex and critically ill of the PE patients pose unique challenges to the established management guidelines due to comorbidities, acute organ failure, and physiologic instability. In this issue of *Critical Care Clinics*, we explore the unique aspects of management of the subset of PE patients requiring ICU care. A special effort was made to include a wide variety of perspectives from many disciplines. The goal of this issue is to help intensivists organize a methodical approach to assess, diagnose, risk-stratify, and treat PE in the ICU. Different articles address treatment algorithms on reperfusion therapies, while others focus on the cardiovascular and pulmonary support of the ICU patient. The

Crit Care Clin 36 (2020) xiii–xiv
https://doi.org/10.1016/j.ccc.2020.04.001
0749-0704/20/© 2020 Published by Elsevier Inc.

criticalcare.theclinics.com

editors of this issue would like to thank all contributors who have shared their knowledge and time to make this multidisciplinary issue of *Critical Care Clinics* come to fruition.

Bharat Awsare, MD
Department of Medicine
Division of Pulmonary and Critical Care
Jefferson University Hospital
Korman Lung Institute
834 Walnut Street, Suite 650
Philadelphia, PA 19107, USA

Michael Baram, MD
Department of Medicine
Division of Pulmonary and Critical Care
Jefferson University Hospital
Korman Lung Institute
834 Walnut Street, Suite 650
Philadelphia, PA 19107, USA

Geno Merli, MD
Department of Medicine and Surgery
Division of Vascular Medicine
Jefferson University Hospital
111 South 11th Street, Suite 6210
Philadelphia, PA 19107, USA

E-mail addresses:
Bharat.Awsare@jefferson.edu (B. Awsare)
Michael.Baram@jefferson.edu (M. Baram)
Geno.Merli@jefferson.edu (G. Merli)

Pulmonary Embolism in Intensive Care Unit

Michael Baram, MD[a],*, Bharat Awsare, MD[a], Geno Merli, MD[b]

KEYWORDS

- Pulmonary embolism (PE) • Intensive care unit • Mortality • Critical care (ICU)
- Massive pulmonary emboli • Submassive pulmonary emboli
- Pulmonary embolism response team (PERT)

KEY POINTS

- Pulmonary embolism continues to have significant morbidity and mortality.
- The management of pulmonary embolism has become more complex due to a proliferation of therapeutic options, requiring communication between multiple specialties in the hospital setting.
- The invention of multidisciplinary teams that are activated helps improve communication, standardize care, and mobilize local resources to manage pulmonary embolism.

INTRODUCTION

Pulmonary embolism (PE) can be a lethal diagnosis, which is often made postmortem.[1–4] The precise morbidity and mortality, however, are difficult to determine due to a variety of presentations, which can vary from prehospital sudden death, death within 24 hours, or death over 1-year follow-up.[1,2,5–7] The mortality from PE is due to acute or progressive right ventricular (RV) failure and may be affected by underlying comorbidities and unintended complications of therapy.[8] Patients are more likely to die of their coexisting cancer, congestive heart failure, or chronic lung disease rather than directly from the PE.[8] The focus of this article is to review the epidemiology, pathophysiology, and natural evolution of disease; the role of the intensive care unit (ICU) in management; and factors that have led to the adoption of PE response teams (PERTs).

EPIDEMIOLOGY OF PULMONARY EMBOLISM

Approximately 1 million to 2 million people in the United States have venous thromboembolisms (VTEs) a year.[2,9,10] The incidence reported by the Centers for Disease

a Department of Medicine, Division of Pulmonary and Critical Care, Jefferson University Hospital, Korman Lung Institute, 834 Walnut Street, Suite 650, Philadelphia, PA 19107, USA; b Department of Medicine and Surgery, Division of Vascular Medicine, Jefferson University Hospital, 111 South 11th Street Suite 6210, Philadelphia, PA 19107, USA
* Corresponding author.
E-mail address: Michael.Baram@jefferson.edu

Crit Care Clin 36 (2020) 427–435
https://doi.org/10.1016/j.ccc.2020.02.001

Control and Prevention is 1 to 2 per 1000 persons per year.[6] The incidence is significantly affected by age, with the rate 1:100,000 in young people and 1:100 in people older than age 80 years.[1,6,10] The rate of new VTE cases increases each decade but accelerates most rapidly during the sixth decade of life.[9–11] It is a disease that affects all races, ethnicities, ages, and genders.[6] PE potentially accounts directly for 3% of all US deaths and indirectly contributes to another 6%.[1] **Fig. 1** displays the scope of VTE problem. Of patients with deep venous thrombosis (DVT), 25% have a progression to symptomatic PE, thus generating a US occurrence rate of 500,000 new PE cases per year.[2,6,12] Based on nationwide hospital admission databases, there are approximately 200,000 annual hospital admissions for PE.[13] An Australian study suggests that PEs causing ICU admission occur in 11 cases per million people per year.[15] Approximately 5% of admitted ICU patients die in the hospital.[13] Of all symptomatic PEs, 20% die prehospital and 5% in hospital, with total of 30% of acute PE patients dying of all-cause mortality within 30 days.[2,8,13] Based on autopsy and extrapolation of databases, approximately 11% of PE deaths occur within the first hour, creating the concept of the golden hour in PE.[1,16] The greatest risk of death occurs within the first 3 months after PE.[8,13] In 2008, the US Surgeon General called attention to the 100,000 to 180,000 US yearly deaths from/with VTE.[9,17] Improved treatment has resulted in lower PE-associated mortality; however, all-cause hospital mortality has increased. This discrepancy is explained by the US national trends to manage some PE patients as outpatients; thus, only higher-acuity patients are admitted.[13] In addition, advances in imaging techniques have diagnosed smaller incidental PEs with low risk stratification, which also contribute to overall lower mortality numbers.[2,12,15]

With an increased effort in DVT prevention, the incidence of ICU-acquired PE has been reported at 1.9%.[9,18,19] The mean time to hospital-acquired PE was 8 days, with hypotension and respiratory distress the 2 most frequent triggers for PE workup.[19,20] This number may be biased by the 10% of patients who may have presented and admitted to the hospital with undiagnosed PE.[20] In brief, patients who have evidence of shock or are at risk of hemodynamic decompensation or massive versus submassive PE frequently are admitted to ICUs.[2,21] Patients at highest risk of deterioration, such as those with moderate to severe RV dysfunction, acute cor pulmonale,

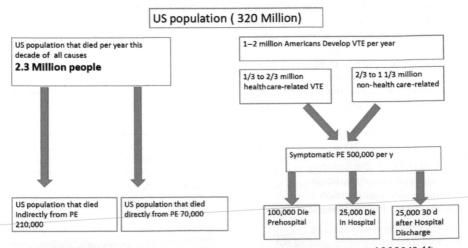

Fig. 1. Yearly incidence of VTEs per year of this decade. (*Data from* Refs.[1,2,6,8,9,12–14])

and clot in transit within the heart, also drive ICU admission.[2] Patients admitted with shock carry a mortality risk of 25% to 50%.[21,22] Patients admitted post–cardiac arrest have a significantly higher mortality of greater than 70%.[23]

The cost of a single PE treatment ranges from $14,000 to $44,000, with the cost of ICU-related PE care presumably higher.[9] The yearly cost of PE treatment is estimated at $2 billion to $10 billion.[6] Preventable VTE could contribute to overall US health care costs of more than $4.5 billion per year.[9] Patients who had VTE either with or without PE had an 80% higher risk of having a disability affecting employment.[24] On average, each first VTE event was associated with an 11-day loss of work.[9] There has been a concerted effort to reduce hospital-acquired VTE to reduce immediate-term and long-term costs from VTE.[18]

PATHOPHYSIOLOGY

PE can be the result of a variety of emboli to the pulmonary artery vasculature from VTEs to air, tumor, amniotic fluid, fat, or foreign bodies, such as coils.[25] Unless mentioned otherwise, the term PE generally refers to VTE. VTE was first reported in thirteenth century reports which documented a probable DVT in the leg of a 20-year-old man with unilateral lower extremity swelling.[10] Theories of why unilateral leg swelling can occur have varied from retention of "evil humors" associated with pregnancy to the accumulation of milk causing thrombosis ("milk leg").[10,26] Rudolf Virchow in 1856 showed that the triad of hypercoagulability, venous stasis, and blood vessel injury predisposed individuals to thrombosis.[2,10,27] There also are environmental/situational, genetic, and modifiable factors that contribute to VTE risk.[6,11,28,29] **Table 1** summarizes some of the more common factors associated with VTE. Adenocarcinoma is the highest risk factor associated with PE.[2] Ramot and colleagues[28] published an extensive review of the literature showing the complex interaction between drugs and their physiologic targets and sometimes unintended consequence of affecting both systemic and venous circulation. Drug effects on VTE can be categorized by their resultant endothelial damage, platelet adhesion or aggregation, white blood cell adhesion, effects on coagulation cascade, and effects on blood flow.[28] Of PE survivors, there is resultant endothelial damage and deconditioning with reduced oxygen consumption that can persist.[30] Approximately 5% of patients are left with residual pulmonary hypertension 90 days postevent.[25,32]

The physiologic effects of a PE remain complex and not fully understood. The clot burden produces mechanical strain by the obstruction, causing increased pulmonary vascular resistance that the thin-walled RV must overcome.[25] Assessment of RV dysfunction is important due to is impact on patient outcome. Clot burden alone, however, does not explain the increased pulmonary vascular resistance and increased RV afterload. For example, there is a significant release of thromboxane A2 and serotonin as a result of the embolic load, which contributes to the vasoconstriction.[25,33] These potent inflammatory mediators have direct local effects and are potential targets of supportive therapy. In addition, the PE causes redistribution of blood flow that can cause ventilation-perfusion (V/Q) mismatch, resulting in regional hypoxia and resulting in further pulmonary vascular vasoconstriction.[34] The resultant RV dilation can cause increased RV wall tension and increased oxygen uptake. When combined with a decreased perfusion pressure, RV ischemia ensues and further decreases RV output and left ventricular (LV) preload. The enlarged RV also can impede LV filling due to ventricular interdependence. The result is a cascade of events leading to RV failure also known as the "right ventricular spiral of death."[25,35]

Table 1		
Risk factor venous thromboembolisms		
Genetic	**Environmental/Situational**	**Lifestyle**
Factor V Leiden	Trauma	Tobacco
Prothrombin G20210A	Orthopedic surgery	Obesity
Protein C or protein S deficiency	Hospitalization (surgery,	Sedentary lifestyle
Antithrombin deficiency	cancer, congestive	Injection drug abuse
Sickle cell	heart failure, COPD)	Long flights
	Medication	
	(contraception,	
	hormone replacement)	
	Obstetrics	
	Indwelling catheters	
	Antiphospholipid syndrome	
	Human immunodeficiency virus	
	Nephrotic syndrome	

Data from Refs.[17,30,31]

ROLE OF THE INTENSIVE CARE UNIT

The ICU is the optimal venue for the monitoring and support of patients with high-risk PE.[15,19,22] There are medical conditions, however, unique to the ICU that make PE management difficult.[36] Diagnostic testing is only positive in 10% to 15% of cases.[36,37] This low yield reflects the nonspecific indications for PE testing (tachycardia and hypoxemia), which are common to the ICU population, as well as the current high testing rates. The positive predictive value of the testing increases as clinical suspicion rises.[25,31,38–40] Intensivists often must function in a model of diagnostic dilemmas while working to stabilize hemodynamics and while trying to confirm a diagnosis—in the paradigm of the golden hour: diagnostic plans and treatment must be succinct.[16,41]

Critical care management of PE includes hemodynamic and oxygen management. Understanding the association of hypoxia, RV afterload, RV failure, and potentially resultant cardiovascular collapse is part of the fundamentals of PE care. The presence of shock and/or cardiac arrest dramatically worsens survival.[16] A more compressive understanding of this high mortality should include the comorbidities associated with or causing PE, the complex interaction of the RV, hypoxia due to V/Q mismatch, and the physiologic reserve.[16,35] Supportive therapies of the RV failure include afterload reduction, inotropic augmentation supported by vasopressors, and fluid management.[16,22] It is essential for intensivists to understand the complex interplay of cardiovascular support and oxygenation support by positive pressure.[42,43] Supportive interventions may be as simple as oxygen supplementation to the extreme of extracorporeal membranous oxygenation (ECMO).[25,44–46] Mortality of mechanically ventilated patients approaches 40%.[15] Patients receiving cardiopulmonary resuscitation have a 65% mortality.[15,47]

THE INTENSIVE CARE UNIT AND MULTIORGAN FAILURE

ICU patients may have multiorgan failure prior to diagnosis of PE, which presents challenges to diagnosis and management of PE, requiring the intensivist to make frequent risk/benefit decisions to treat these patients. Sometimes a diagnosis of VTE is made incidentally, and VTE is not the condition making the patient critically ill.[48] The following is a sample of some unique issues in an ICU that increase the challenges in treating PE.

Central nervous system[49]
- Delirium: inability to cooperate for imaging
- Intracranial hemorrhage or subdural hematoma from trauma complicating therapy for PE

Endocrinopathy[50]
- Tachycardia may mimic PE
- Iodine for computed tomography scan could exacerbate thyroid toxicosis

Pulmonary[51]
- Underlying chronic obstructive pulmonary disease (COPD), asthma, and interstitial lung disease may mimic PE or magnify the effects of PE
- Mechanical ventilation may worsen hemodynamics due to increased RV afterload
- Severe hypoxemia may increase risk of transport for diagnostic imaging

Cardiovascular[40,52]
- Underlying cardiomyopathy, chronic VTE, sleep apnea, and pulmonary hypertension can magnify the effects of PE
- Hemodynamic instability may increase risk of transport for diagnostic imaging
- McConnell sign is not specific for PE and can be found in other causes of RV failure seen in the ICU (RV infarct, acute RV, and dysfunction of mechanical ventilation)
- Antiplatelet agents increase risk of bleeding
- Inferior vena cava filters affect ability to cannulate femoral vein for ECMO

Gastrointestinal[53]
- Gastrointestinal bleeding occurring or recurring with anticoagulation
- Safety of esophagogastroduodenoscopy in setting of PE and gastrointestinal bleeding[51]

Liver failure[54,55]
- Pharmacokinetics of clearance of warfarin or other novel oral anticoagulants
- Persistent state of disseminated intravascular coagulation
- Often with misbalance of coagulation factors, making prothrombin time less reliable as a marker of bleeding risk
- Coagulation factor deficiency due to decreased production
- Chronic liver disease and coagulopathy from malnutrition (vitamin K deficiency)
- Potential for life-threatening variceal bleeding
- Dysfibrinogenemia

Renal failure[56]
- Use of intravenous dye may be limited for diagnostic testing
- Renal clearance of drugs (direct oral anticoagulant, heparin, and low-molecular-weight heparin)

Hematologic
- Risk of bleeding with thrombocytopenia
- Risk of heparin-induced thrombocytopenia
- Severe anemia can reduce effectiveness of fibrin deposition to stop bleeding
- Antiphospholipid syndrome
- Hypercoagulable states associated with malignancy

Postoperative patients/trauma patients
- Increased bleeding risk

PULMONARY EMBOLISM RESPONSE TEAMS

Over the past decade, there have been increasing options for acute PE care. These include novel anticoagulants; catheter-directed therapies; RV support systems, such as venoarterial ECMO and RV assist devices; alternate dosing of systemic thrombolytics; and a renewed interest in surgical embolectomy.[22] In response to this, PERTs have formed to facilitate decision making.[2,16,57] Some of the common constituents of a PERT team include pulmonary/critical care, vascular medicine, interventional radiology, hematology, cardiology, emergency medicine, and cardiothoracic surgery.[58] Each institution has different resources and varying levels of expertise that necessitate unique institutional algorithms of care.

Similar to how tumor boards have improved the standardization and quality of cancer care, the PERT model hopes to achieve the same goals with PE.[59] The PERT can conference at the bedside or virtually using modern communication technology. Data, such as imaging, risk stratification, and availability of interventions, can be shared among team members.[59] Team decision making can help reduce errors and may support interventions that are more aggressive yet potentially beneficial.[57,60] Literature suggests that there is an underutilization of PE interventions, such as systemic thrombolytics in massive PE, despite growing evidence.[60] PERT teams that have published their data have shown increase utilization of various reperfusion techniques over time without increase in bleeding complication.[57]

SUMMARY

With the increasing complexity of health care delivery, the ICU will continue to play a pivotal role of PE management. Fortunately, the formation of PERT teams has increased the resources available to care for these critically ill patients. The remainder of the issue elaborates on the diagnostics, therapeutic, and multidisciplinary management topics raised in this introduction and provides intensivists a greater knowledge of the principles necessary in the management of high-risk PE.

DISCLOSURE

All authors have nothing to disclose.

REFERENCES

1. Dalen JE, Alpert JS. Natural history of pulmonary embolism. Prog Cardiovasc Dis 1975;17(4):259–70.
2. Giordano NJ, Jansson PS, Young MN, et al. Epidemiology, pathophysiology, stratification, and natural history of pulmonary embolism. Tech Vasc Interv Radiol 2017;20(3):135–40.
3. Barnes AR. Pulmonary embolism. J Am Med Assoc 1937;109(17):1347–53.
4. Phear D. Pulmonary embolism: a study of late prognosis. Lancet 1960;276(7155): 832–5.
5. Kirch W, Schafii C. Misdiagnosis at a university hospital in 4 medical eras. Medicine (Baltimore) 1996;75(1):29–40.
6. Beckman MG, Hooper WC, Critchley SE, et al. Venous thromboembolism: a public health concern. Am J Prev Med 2010;38(4 Suppl):S495–501.
7. Goldman L, Sayson R, Robbins S, et al. The value of the autopsy in three medical eras. N Engl J Med 1983;308(17):1000–5.
8. Carson JL, Kelley MA, Duff A, et al. The clinical course of pulmonary embolism. N Engl J Med 1992;326(19):1240–5.
9. Mahan CE, Borrego ME, Woersching AL, et al. Venous thromboembolism: annualised United States models for total, hospital-acquired and preventable costs utilising long-term attack rates. Thromb Haemost 2012;108(2):291–302.

10. Lijfering WM, Rosendaal FR, Cannegieter SC. Risk factors for venous thrombosis - current understanding from an epidemiological point of view. Br J Haematol 2010;149(6):824–33.

11. Goldhaber SZ. Risk factors for venous thromboembolism. J Am Coll Cardiol 2010; 56(1):1–7.

12. Anderson FA, Zayaruzny M, Heit JA, et al. Estimated annual numbers of US acute-care hospital patients at risk for venous thromboembolism. Am J Hematol 2007;82(9):777–82.

13. Smith SB, Geske JB, Kathuria P, et al. Analysis of national trends in admissions for pulmonary embolism. Chest 2016;150(1):35–45.

14. Spencer FA, Lessard D, Emery C, et al. Venous thromboembolism in the outpatient setting. Arch Intern Med 2007;167(14):1471–5.

15. Winterton D, Bailey M, Pilcher D, et al. Characteristics, incidence and outcome of patients admitted to intensive care because of pulmonary embolism. Respirology 2017;22(2):329–37.

16. Wood KE. Major pulmonary embolism: review of a pathophysiologic approach to the golden hour of hemodynamically significant pulmonary embolism. Chest 2002;121(3):877–905.

17. Office of the Surgeon General (US); National Heart, Lung, and Blood Institute (US). The Surgeon General's call to action to prevent deep vein thrombosis and pulmonary embolism. Rockville (MD): Office of the Surgeon General (US); 2008. Available from: https://www.ncbi.nlm.nih.gov/books/NBK44178/.

18. Clagett GP, Anderson FA, Geerts W, et al. Prevention of venous thromboembolism. Chest 1998;114(5 Suppl):531S–60S.

19. Bahloul M, Chaari A, Kallel H, et al. Pulmonary embolism in intensive care unit: predictive factors, clinical manifestations and outcome. Ann Thorac Med 2010; 5(2):97–103.

20. Attia J, Ray JG, Cook DJ, et al. Deep vein thrombosis and its prevention in critically ill adults. Arch Intern Med 2001;161(10):1268–79.

21. Kearon C. Natural history of venous thromboembolism. Circulation 2003;107(23 Suppl 1):I22–30.

22. Marshall PS, Mathews KS, Siegel MD. Diagnosis and management of life-threatening pulmonary embolism. J Intensive Care Med 2011;26(5):275–94.

23. Kurkciyan I, Meron G, Sterz F, et al. Pulmonary embolism as a cause of cardiac arrest: presentation and outcome. Arch Intern Med 2000;160(10):1529–35.

24. Braekkan SK, Grosse SD, Okoroh EM, et al. Venous thromboembolism and subsequent permanent work-related disability. J Thromb Haemost 2016;14(10): 1978–87.

25. Essien EO, Rali P, Mathai SC. Pulmonary embolism. Med Clin North Am 2019; 103(3):549–64.

26. Mannucci PM. Venous thrombosis: the history of knowledge. Pathophysiol Haemost Thromb 2002;32(5–6):209–12.

27. Virchow R. *Phlogose und Thrombose im Gefäßsystem.Gesammelte Abhandlungen zur wissenschaftlichen Medicin.* Gesammelte Abhandlungen zur wissenschaftlichen Medicin. Berlin: von Meiniger; 1856.

28. Ramot Y, Nyska A, Spectre G. Drug-induced thrombosis: an update. Drug Saf 2013;36(8):585–603.

29. Connors JM. Thrombophilia testing and venous thrombosis. N Engl J Med 2017; 377(12):1177–87.

30. Albaghdadi MS, Dudzinski DM, Giordano N, et al. Cardiopulmonary exercise testing in patients following massive and submassive pulmonary embolism. J Am Heart Assoc 2018;7(5) [pii:e006841].
31. Anderson FA Jr, Spencer FA. Risk factors for venous thromboembolism. Circulation 2003;107(23 Suppl 1):I9–16.
32. Ribeiro A, Lindmarker P, Johnsson H, et al. Pulmonary embolism: one-year follow-up with echocardiography Doppler and five-year survival analysis. Circulation 1999;99(10):1325–30.
33. Smulders Y. Pathophysiology and treatment of haemodynamic instability in acute pulmonary embolism: the pivotal role of pulmonary vasoconstriction. Cardiovasc Res 2000;48(1):23–33.
34. Altemeier WA, Robertson HT, McKinney S, et al. Pulmonary embolization causes hypoxemia by redistributing regional blood flow without changing ventilation. J Appl Physiol (1985) 1998;85(6):2337–43.
35. Matthews JC, McLaughlin V. Acute right ventricular failure in the setting of acute pulmonary embolism or chronic pulmonary hypertension: a detailed review of the pathophysiology, diagnosis, and management. Curr Cardiol Rev 2008;4(1): 49–59.
36. Konstantinides SV, Torbicki A, Agnelli G, et al. 2014 ESC guidelines on the diagnosis and management of acute pulmonary embolism. Eur Heart J 2014;35(43): 3033–69.
37. McFarlane MJ, Imperiale TF. Use of the alveolar-arterial oxygen gradient in the diagnosis of pulmonary embolism. Am J Med 1994;96(1):57–62.
38. Investigators P. Value of the ventilation/perfusion scan in acute pulmonary embolism. Results of the prospective investigation of pulmonary embolism diagnosis (PIOPED). JAMA 1990;263(20):2753–9.
39. Worsley DF, Alavi A, Comprehensive analysis of the results of the PIOPED study. Prospective investigation of pulmonary embolism diagnosis study. J Nucl Med 1995;36(12):2380–7.
40. Vaid U, Singer E, Marhefka G, et al. Poor positive predictive value of McConnell's sign on transthoracic echocardiography for the diagnosis of acute pulmonary embolism. Hosp Pract (1995) 2013;41(3):23–7.
41. Marini JJ. Re-tooling critical care to become a better intensivist: something old and something new. Crit Care 2015;19(Suppl 3):S3.
42. Marik PE, Baram M. Noninvasive hemodynamic monitoring in the intensive care unit. Crit Care Clin 2007;23(3):383–400.
43. Khemasuwan D, Yingchoncharoen T, Tunsupon P, et al. Right ventricular echocardiographic parameters are associated with mortality after acute pulmonary embolism. J Am Soc Echocardiogr 2015;28(3):355–62.
44. Awsare B, Herman J, Baram M. Management strategies for severe respiratory failure: as extracorporeal membrane oxygenation is being considered. Crit Care Clin 2017;33(4):795–811.
45. Wong JK, Siow V, Hirose H, et al. End organ recovery and survival with the QuadroxD Oxygenator in adults on extracorporeal membran oxygenation. World J Cardiovasc Surg 2012;2(04):73–80.
46. Slottosch I, Liakopoulos O, Kuhn E, et al. Lactate and lactate clearance as valuable tool to evaluate ECMO therapy in cardiogenic shock. J Crit Care 2017;42: 35–41.
47. Kasper W, Konstantinides S, Geibel A, et al. Management strategies and determinants of outcome in acute major pulmonary embolism: results of a multicenter registry. J Am Coll Cardiol 1997;30(5):1165–71.

48. O'Connell C. Incidentally found pulmonary embolism: what's the clinician to do? Hematol Am Soc Hematol Educ Program 2015;2015:197–201.
49. Chatterjee S, Weinberg I, Yeh RW, et al. Risk factors for intracranial haemorrhage in patients with pulmonary embolism treated with thrombolytic therapy Development of the PE-CH Score. Thromb Haemost 2017;117(2):246–51.
50. Segna D, Mean M, Limacher A, et al. Association between thyroid dysfunction and venous thromboembolism in the elderly: a prospective cohort study. J Thromb Haemost 2016;14(4):685–94.
51. Moua T, Wood K. COPD and PE: a clinical dilemma. Int J Chron Obstruct Pulmon Dis 2008;3(2):277–84.
52. Friedman O, Horowitz JM, Ramzy D. Advanced cardiopulmonary support for pulmonary embolism. Tech Vasc Interv Radiol 2017;20(3):179–84.
53. Radaelli F, Dentali F, Repici A, et al. Management of anticoagulation in patients with acute gastrointestinal bleeding. Dig Liver Dis 2015;47(8):621–7.
54. Amitrano L, Guardascione M, Brancaccio V, et al. Coagulation disorders in liver disease. Semin Liver Dis 2002;22(1):83–96.
55. Qamar A, Vaduganathan M, Greenberger N, et al. Oral anticoagulation in patients with liver disease. J Am Coll Cardiol 2018;71(19):2162–75.
56. Grand'Maison A, Charest AF, Geerts WH. Anticoagulant use in patients with chronic renal impairment. Am J Cardiovasc Drugs 2005;5(5):291–305.
57. Kabrhel C, Rosovsky R, Channick R, et al. A multidisciplinary pulmonary embolism response team: initial 30-month experience with a novel approach to delivery of care to patients with submassive and massive pulmonary embolism. Chest 2016;150(2):384–93.
58. Rodriguez-Lopez J, Channick R. The pulmonary embolism response team: what is the ideal model? Semin Respir Crit Care Med 2017;38(1):51–5.
59. Nallamothu BK, Cohen DJ. No "i" in Heart Team: incentivizing multidisciplinary care in cardiovascular medicine. Circ Cardiovasc Qual Outcomes 2012;5(3):410–3.
60. Galie N, Manes A, Dardi F, et al. Thrombolysis in high-risk patients with acute pulmonary embolism: underuse of a life-saving treatment in the real-world setting. Eur Heart J 2019;41(4):530–3.

Risk Stratification of Pulmonary Embolism

Thomas Moumneh, MD[a,b,c], Philip S. Wells, MD, FRCP(C), MSc[d],*,
Sebastien Miranda, MD[c,e,f]

KEYWORDS

- Pulmonary embolism • Risk stratification • Prognosis • Mortality • Biomarkers
- Clinical assessment

KEY POINTS

- Patients diagnosed with pulmonary embolism who survived cardiac arrest or presented in shock have poor outcomes and should receive pharmacoinvasive treatments.
- Various combinations of clinical parameters, biomarkers and imaging may provide reasonable estimates of the risk of death in the first 30 days.
- The available literature on prognosis of pulmonary embolism is limited by a nonstandardized definition of pulmonary embolism-related death and a failure to consider competing risks for death.
- To date, no study has demonstrated an improvement in mortality rates after implementation of a risk stratification strategy to guide treatment.
- Many studies evaluating prognostic tools have failed to use proper methodologic design.

INTRODUCTION

Risk stratification of pulmonary embolism (PE) is a challenging but desirable component of PE management. Given the broad treatment options, ranging from urgent thrombectomy to no treatment, and the choice of sending the patient to urgent surgery or intensive care monitoring, or discharging for ambulatory management, risk stratification is important. Currently available treatments are very effective once begun, with a residual risk of dying from PE of less than 1.5% in observational registries.[1,2]

---

[a] Department of Emergency Medicine, University Hospital of Angers, 4 rue Larrey, 49100 Angers, France; [b] MITOVASC Institute, UMR CNRS 6015 UMR INSERM 1083, Angers University, 28, rue Roger-Amsler, 49045 Angers, France; [c] University of Ottawa, 451 Smyth Road, Ottawa, Ontario, Canada; [d] Department of Medicine, University of Ottawa, Ottawa Hospital Research Institute, 501 Smyth Road, Suite M1857, PO Box 206, Ottawa, Ontario K1H 8L6, Canada; [e] Department of Internal Medicine, Vascular and Thrombosis Unit, Rouen University Hospital, 37 Boulevard Gambetta, 76000 Rouen, France; [f] Normandie University, UNIROUEN, INSERM U1096, 22 Boulevard Gambetta, 76000 Rouen, France
* Corresponding author.
E-mail address: pwells@toh.ca

Crit Care Clin 36 (2020) 437–448
https://doi.org/10.1016/j.ccc.2020.02.002
0749-0704/20/© 2020 Elsevier Inc. All rights reserved.

criticalcare.theclinics.com

It is even more challenging if the physician must risk stratify patients before the diagnosis of PE is confirmed, such as in the case of patients who are not sufficiently stable to receive conclusive imaging.[3] However, because presentation with cardiac arrest owing to PE is associated with a greater than 80% in-hospital mortality, patients with such a severe PE do not need further risk stratification.[3,4] Similarly, shock, a systolic blood pressure less than 90 mm Hg or a pressure decrease of 40 mm Hg or more for longer than 15 minutes if not caused by new-onset arrythmias, hypovolemia, or sepsis has a high risk of death[3,5]; thrombolysis or thrombectomy are the treatment choices, chosen based on local expertise and resources.

Data suggest that, without appropriate treatment, the risk for death from PE is substantial, but it is not easy to precisely estimate this risk.[6,7] Submassive PE that leads to right ventricular dysfunction may cause death, but death may also be related to myocardial infarction, respiratory failure from impaired gas exchange, hemoptysis related to pulmonary infarction, or even complications from the treatment such as hemorrhage.[8] As such, risk stratification may depend on clot burden, but also on baseline cardiopulmonary function, other comorbidities, risk of recurrent emboli and efficacy or harm from treatment. These competing factors emphasize the need to determine whether the risk of death acutely is due to the presenting PE per se and thus potentially preventable. Similarly, death after the acute phase of treatment may be due to the recurrence of the PE after seemingly appropriate treatment has been initiated, or because of other issues such as terminal cancer or end-stage chronic obstructive pulmonary disease. Unfortunately, proving death has occurred specifically because of the PE is problematic. Challenges in the definition and identification of PE-caused death are such that the surrogate of death from any cause is typical in studies of prognosis.[7,9] Most patients experiencing death after being diagnosed with PE have underlying diseases that are associated with a significant risk of death independent of the PE.[10] Even the use of central adjudication to determine if death is PE related is currently of limited benefit because this process has been shown to be imprecise and poorly reproducible.[11] Post mortem computed tomographic pulmonary angiography (CTPA) is unable to opacify pulmonary arteries and consequently not useful in identifying fatal PE.[12] The reference standard for a fatal PE diagnosis perhaps would be systematic necropsy, but even this costly and unfeasible approach does not prove causality; the criteria to diagnose PE-related death on necropsy are not well-established. These limitations emphasize the importance of randomized trials that compare interventions with patients selected based on having a proven prognostic factor.

As an aside, it is worth noting that many deaths from PE are likely a result of failure to suspect PE and promptly initiate treatment. Some authors demonstrated worse outcomes in patients in whom diagnose was delayed.[13,14] In addition, it seems that PE was not suspected in many fatal PE confirmed on necropsy.[7,15,16] But, apart from increasing awareness on the need to suspect PE and to initiate appropriate treatment early, PE suspicion is a topic we do not address in this article.

Taking into consideration these limitations, this review strives to generate hypotheses regarding prognostic factors able to predict death in patients with PE, with the caveat that we cannot conclude death is due to PE. This limitation will be implicit in our conclusions on each prognostic factor discussed.

CLOT BURDEN

The belief that the amount of thrombus correlates with higher risk of death may seem logical, but the biological and radiologic markers of clot burden are not necessarily related to the risk of death. We first discuss the direct quantification of clot in the lung through imaging, and then indirect quantification of clot burden by lower extremity venous ultrasound examination and D-dimer levels.

Computed Tomographic Pulmonary Angiography

Direct assessment of arterial obstruction was historically assessed with intravenous contrast pulmonary artery angiography. CTPA has replaced this procedure and, along with lung perfusion scintigraphy, can provide reliable estimates of obstruction when compared with the gold standard.[17] The importance of obstruction may be related to location especially for central, so-called saddle PE, but may best be estimated by obstruction indices that were created to reflect the total vascular obstruction (eg, the Mastora, Qanadli, or Meyer score).[17–19] Correlation between these scores and the clinical severity and outcome of the PE was initially suspected, but a meta-analysis published in 2013 showed a weak association with the risk of death at 30 days and a concerning heterogeneity.[20] Within the same meta-analysis, identification of a thrombus within the proximal pulmonary arteries was inconsistently associated with the 30-day risk of death.

More recently, retrospective matched cohorts of patients with saddle versus non-saddle PE showed no difference in short term (<6 hours) or in-hospital mortality after PE diagnosis.[21,22] Thus, neither obstruction index nor location of PE in hemodynamically stable patients have the capacity to guide the use of thrombolytics or embolectomy.

Transthoracic Echocardiography

The visualization of the thrombus on transthoracic echocardiography is a dramatic finding. A meta-analysis of 6 studies demonstrated a 3.0-fold increased risk of death by 30 days compared with patients without evidence of right ventricular thrombus.[23] However, these results are biased by the absence of adjustment for the hemodynamic status of the patient. Therefore, visualization of thrombus on transesophageal echocardiography is useful for diagnosis, but it has not been proven that the identification of an intracardiac thrombus is helpful to determine risk and to guide treatment. Indeed, the same authors found no difference in mortality comparing thrombolysis with anticoagulants, but statistically fewer recurrences occurred in the anticoagulation group.[24]

Lower Extremity Venous Ultrasonography

Documenting concomitant deep vein thrombosis (DVT) that could embolize and destabilize the hemodynamic status could be helpful. A meta-analysis published in 2016 found an association between the presence of concomitant DVT and 30-day mortality in patients with acute PE (odds ratio [OR] 1.89; 95% confidence interval [CI], 1.52–2.36), but the positive predictive value of lower extremity venous ultrasound examination to predict early mortality was only 6.2%.[25] Moreover, a prospective randomized controlled trial (PREPIC) demonstrated that systematic insertion of an inferior vena cava filter in patients with acute PE with concomitant DVT and risk factors for recurrence did not prevent mortality or recurrence.[26]

D-Dimers

Apart from visualization of the thrombus, measurement of the D-dimer level is suggested to be related to the clot burden and right ventricular dysfunction.[27–29] In a meta-analysis based on 22 studies, 5 studies (2885 patients) evaluated the correlation between short-term mortality and D-dimer levels (in-hospital or 15-day mortality in 4 studies, 30-day mortality in 1 study).[30] Patients with levels above the prognostic cut-offs had a higher risk of short-term mortality (OR, 2.76; 95% CI, 1.83–4.14).

However, these results may be of limited relevance because the studies used different cut-off values and different D-dimer assays.

CLINICAL PARAMETERS

Syncope

Syncope associated with PE is concerning because an embolus large enough to briefly compromise cerebral perfusion (a presumed mechanism of the syncope) may continue to compromise circulation. A recent meta-analysis of 28 studies found a significant association between syncope and 30-day mortality (OR, 1.73; 95% CI, 1.22–2.47).[31] However, there was a strong association between hemodynamic instability and presentation with syncope. When restricting the meta-analysis to only hemodynamically stable patients, syncope was not associated with in-hospital mortality (OR, 0.50; 95% CI, 0.18–1.43) or 30-day mortality (OR, 1.09; 95% CI, 0.55–2.16). This finding suggests that only hemodynamic instability reliably predicts risk of death. Syncope should not be considered an independent marker of mortality.

Hypotension

Hypotension is rarely present in acute PE, recently estimated at 3.9% in more than 40,000 patients with new PE.[5] Obviously, patients in hemodynamic collapse have a worse prognosis, but surprisingly there are limited data to support this notion. In a recently published meta-analysis of 4 cohorts of consecutive patient with PE, those with hemodynamic instability had an OR of 5.9 (95% CI, 2.7–13.0) for all-cause mortality in first 90 days.[5] A prospective study of more than 1300 patients determined true short-term (1-week) mortality was significantly increased (OR, 3.35; 95% CI, 1.51–5.41) in patients who initially presented with systolic arterial hypotension, defined as a blood pressure of greater than 100 mm Hg, or immobilization owing to a medical illness (OR, 2.89; 95% CI, 1.31–6.39).[32] Hemodynamic instability remains the only widely agreed upon indication for thrombolysis,[8,33] based on the 50% decrease in the mortality rate in an earlier study.[34]

Hemoptysis

Hemoptysis is a relatively rare presentation for PE.[35] To our knowledge, no studies have described an increased risk of death associated with hemoptysis. Hemoptysis related to PE is mostly related to pulmonary infarction and is unlikely to result in a fatal hemorrhage.

Clinical Scores

Numerous rules based on clinical data have been developed to stratify risk in patients with PE. The best known are the Pulmonary Embolism Severity Index (PESI) score, the simplified Pulmonary Embolism Severity Index (sPESI), the Hestia criteria, and the Geneva prognostic score.

The Pulmonary Embolism Severity Index and simplified Pulmonary Embolism Severity Index

The PESI was originally derived from a large retrospective registry of patients diagnosed with PE, to predict 30-day mortality. It includes 11 clinical criteria and classifies patients in up to 5 categories of risk, ranging from a 90-day mortality of 0% in the very low-risk group to 18% in the very high-risk group.[36] Because it predicts all-cause mortality, it is not surprising to find age and cancer as leading predictors. The PESI was later simplified—the sPESI. It includes 6 items, identically weighted. It was validated and shown to be as accurate as the original PESI.[37] It was later implemented and used to selected patients suitable for outpatient management. Patients meeting none of the sPESI items were shown to have a very low risk of death with home management of PE. It has also been used in association with biomarkers and imaging studies to further assess patients at risk for mortality.[8,38]

The Hestia criteria
The Hestia criteria is a checklist of situations that, when present, are supposed to contraindicate ambulatory treatment of newly diagnosed PE. They do not correspond with a severity score, but mortality during follow-up has been studied. In patients meeting none of the Hestia criteria, the risk of all-cause mortality is very low.[39] Meeting 1 or more of the Hestia criteria has been recommended as indicating a need for inpatient management, but this metric does not further risk stratify patients and has not been tested in a randomized trial.

The Geneva prognostic score
Using the items of the original Geneva score, a prognostic risk assessment model was derived to predict adverse outcomes in patients diagnosed with PE.[40] Adverse events comprise not only death, but major bleeding and recurrent venous thromboembolism. It includes 6 items but is less practical than the sPESI because it requires proximal leg vein ultrasound examination and an arterial blood sample in the calculation. External validation studies are few. Interestingly, a history of DVT and/or presence of a proximal DVT were found to be independently associated with the risk of serious adverse events, although the association was weak. The other clinical items are all part of the PESI score.

MARKERS OF RIGHT VENTRICULAR DYSFUNCTION
Biomarkers

Cardiac troponin
Cardiac troponin is a very specific of myocardial injury and is mainly used for diagnosis of acute myocardial infarction. However, troponin was also shown to predict mortality in patients assessed for acute myocardial infarction, but ultimately not diagnosed with an acute myocardial infarction.[41,42] In the context of PE, cardiac troponin elevation likely reflects right ventricular dysfunction. Troponin was shown to be a rather specific biomarker of right ventricular dysfunction in the context of PE, but not very sensitive.[43] Several meta-analyses have suggested elevated troponins predict 30-day all-cause mortality. Most recently a meta-analysis found early all-cause mortality rates, based on elevated troponins, of 3.8% (95% CI, 2.1%–6.8%) versus 0.5% (95% CI, 0.2%–1.3%) for normal levels for an OR of 6.25 (95% CI, 1.95–20.05).[44] There are many troponin measurement assays commercially available, with various levels indicating an abnormal result. These so-called cut-off points or thresholds were developed in patients suspected to have acute coronary syndromes and validated in this context. Most studies used those same thresholds in patients with PE to determine the level that indicates right ventricular dysfunction. Some studies suggest an exponential increase in the risk of inpatient all-cause mortality in association with the troponin level.[45]

Brain natriuretic peptide and N-terminal pro b-type natriuretic peptide
Brain natriuretic peptides (BNPs) are secreted by cardiomyocytes in response to stretching, and therefore it is logical levels will increase in the context of right ventricular dysfunction related to PE. As opposed to troponin, BNP and/or N-terminal pro b-type natriuretic peptide are more sensitive than specific for right ventricular dysfunction.[43] An increased risk of early PE-related mortality was reported in recent meta-

analysis, with a rate of 1.7% (95% CI, 0.4%–6.9%) in the elevated BNP group versus 0.4% (95% CI, 0.1%–1.1%) in the normal BNP group, for an OR of 3.71 (95% CI, 0.81–17.02).[44] Decision thresholds vary widely across studies, from 21.7 to 100 pg/mL for BNP, and from 300 to 1000 pg/mL for N-terminal pro b-type natriuretic peptide.

Heart-type fatty acid-binding protein

Heart-type fatty acid-binding protein (H-FABP) is a protein widely expressed in cardiomyocytes and released in the context of an acute coronary syndrome. A meta-analysis of 11 small studies found an increased 30-day PE-related mortality with an OR of 26 (95% CI, 6.6–102) in hemodynamically stable patients. They also found increased risk of a complicated clinical course, defined as all-cause death, need for thrombolytics, endotracheal intubation, catecholamine infusion for sustained hypotension, cardiopulmonary resuscitation, or recurrent PE (OR, 12; 95% CI, 4.1–35.0).[46] There are no head-to-head comparisons between H-FABP and troponin/BNP, but in a meta-analysis H-FABP had better performances than the other biomarkers in predicting 30-day PE-related mortality.[47] Thresholds used for decision were consistent among studies (6–7 ng/mL), but to date H-FABP has not been widely implemented.

Electrocardiography

The electrocardiogram is a readily available and inexpensive tool that may provide indirect information about increased pulmonary artery pressure and right ventricular dysfunction.[48] A meta-analysis based on 10 studies totaling 3007 patients demonstrated the following electrocardiogram findings were associated with an increased risk of hemodynamic collapse or death: sinus tachycardia of greater than 100 beats/min (OR, 4.46; 95% CI, 1.68–11.84), complete right bundle branch block (OR, 2.67; 95% CI, 1.81–3.95), S1Q3T3 (OR, 2.06; 95% CI, 1.23–3.45), and ST elevation in lead aVR (OR, 5.24; 95% CI, 3.98–6.91.)[49] However, these findings were more frequently present in patients with shock at presentation. To our knowledge, no study has prospectively demonstrated that electrocardiogram abnormalities can reliably define a high-risk subgroup.

Transthoracic Echocardiogram

Transthoracic echocardiography demonstrates that right ventricular dysfunction is not uncommon, occurring in 27% to 55% of normotensive patients.[3,50–52] The most common echocardiographic findings in acute PE are a right ventricular end-diastolic diameter of greater than 30 mm, a right ventricular/left ventricular end-diastolic diameter of greater than 1, or right ventricular hypokinesia. Other criteria included paradoxic septal wall motion, pulmonary hypertension, and severe tricuspid regurgitation. A meta-analysis of prospective and retrospective studies suggested potential usefulness. In the prospective study subgroup of this meta-analysis, patients with right ventricular dysfunction by echocardiogram had a 1.61-fold increase in short-term mortality.[53]

Computed Tomographic Pulmonary Angiography

In 1 meta-analysis patients with acute PE with a right ventricular/left ventricular diameter ratio of 1.0 or greater measured on transverse sections by CTPA had a 2.5-fold increased risk for all-cause mortality (OR, 2.5; 95% CI, 1.8–3.5) and a 5-fold risk for PE-related mortality (OR, 5.0; 95% CI, 2.7–9.2).[54] However, studies were included regardless of quality, many studies were retrospective, and the incremental prognostic value of CTPA over clinical and biomarker factors was not assessed. In addition, the difficulty of determining PE-related death was not addressed in this analysis.

Combination of Clinical, Biomarker, and Imaging Findings

Some strategies have tried to associate clinical and nonclinical factors to further risk stratify patients with stable PE. The combination of biomarkers (troponin and/or BNP) and radiologic evidence of right ventricular dysfunction was shown to modestly improved risk stratification when combined with sPESI score.[55] The presence of evidence of right ventricular dysfunction by biomarkers and imaging was shown to be

Table 1
Odds ratio of short-term all-cause mortality based on the presence of prognosis factors in patients with acute PE

	30 d Mortality: OR (95% CI)	Reference
Clot burden		
CTPA obstruction index proximal	1.78 (1.08–2.93)	Vedovati et al,[20] 2013
Intracardiac thrombus transthoracic echocardiography	3.03 (2.24–4.11)	Barrios et al,[23] 2017
DVT on extremity US ELEVATED	1.89 (1.52–2.36)	Becattini et al,[25] 2016
D-Dimer	2.76 (1.83–4.14)	Becattini et al,[30] 2012
Clinical parameters		
Hypotension	3.35 (1.51–5.41)[c]	Conget et al,[32] 2008
Syncope		Barco et al,[31] 2018
All patients	1.73 (1.22–2.47)	
Hemodynamically stable	1.09 (0.55–2.16)	
Hemoptysis	NA	-
sPESI[b]		Zhou et al,[37] 2012
0 point	1% (0–2.1)	
>1 point	10.9% (8.5%-13.2%)	
Right ventricular dysfunction/injury		
Troponin	6.25 (1.95–20.05)	Barco et al,[44] 2019
BNP	3.71 (0.81–17.02)	Barco et al,[44] 2019
H-FABP	26 (6.6–102)	Bajaj et al,[46] 2015
Transthoracic echocardiography		Cho et al,[53] 2014
Electrocardiogram[a]		Shopp et al,[49] 2015
Heart rate >100 bpm	4.46 (1.68–11.84)	
S1Q3T3	2.06 (1.23–3.45)	
Complete right bundle branch block	2.67 (1.81–3.95)	
ST elevation aVR	5.24 (3.98–6.91)	
CTPA	2.5 (1.8–3.5)	Meinel et al.[54] 2015

These results should be carefully be interpreted because rate of patients with hemodynamic collapse was different within the studies and endpoint was not predefined in all studies used for the metanalysis.

Abbreviations: DVT, deep vein thrombosis; US, ultrasound.

[a] Odds ratios for the electrocardiogram components for the risk of hemodynamic collapse or death.

[b] Results expressed in percent risk of mortality at 30 days.

[c] Mortality in the first week.

associated with worse outcomes.[38] Another study, combining individual data from 4 prospective studies of 2874 stable patients diagnosed with PE, found 4 factors to be independently associated with 30-day definite PE-related death, unexplained death, hemodynamic collapse, or recurrent PE.[56] These factors were blood pressure between 90 and 100 mm Hg, a heart rate of 110 beats per minute or more, elevated cardiac troponins, or evidence of right ventricular dysfunction on CTPA or echocardiogram. They developed a risk score, called the Bova score, with 3 risk categories. The first category classified 75% of patients with PE with a 30-day PE-related mortality rate of 1.7%. The second had a 5% mortality rate, and the third, comprising 6% of patients, had a 15.5% PE-related mortality rate to 30 days and a 28% in-hospital PE-related complication rate (composite outcome of PE-related death, hemodynamic collapse, and recurrent nonfatal PE). Later, external validation showed the Bova score showed no significant improvement in comparison with combination of sPESI score and evidence of right ventricular dysfunction.[57]

SUMMARY

Although research in this area suffers from methodical flaws that cast doubt on the validity of the data there are many studies and it seems that numerous clinical parameters, imaging tests, and biomarkers have the potential to prognosticate all-cause mortality in patients with PE. It seems in particular that various combinations of clinical parameters, biomarkers, and imaging may provide reasonable estimates of the risk of death in the first 30 days. Prediction of risk of death in the truly acute phase—that is, the first week of treatment—has not been as well-researched. Regardless, for prediction of death to be clinically useful, intervention studies must demonstrate there is value in such determinations. The PEITHO trial compared systemic thrombolysis versus placebo in hemodynamically stable patients with PE. The study selected patients with right ventricular injury based on cardiac imaging (transthoracic echocardiography or CTPA, and troponin elevation) and demonstrated statistically significantly lower rates of a combined outcome of death or hemodynamic decompensation with thrombolysis, but not a decrease in death as a single outcome. Furthermore, thrombolysis was associated with significantly more strokes, in particular hemorrhagic strokes.[58] Thus, systemic thrombolytic therapy is not recommended for hemodynamically stable patients and the therapeutic implication of risk stratification using these criteria remains limited.[8,33] The PEITHO III trial will test a reduced dose of thrombolytic treatment for patients with intermediate high-risk PE based on these criteria.

Moreover, PE-related mortality is more difficult to predict and intervention studies, based on using prognostic markers, have not demonstrated advantages measured as a decrease in mortality by a priori knowledge of mortality risk. A potential cause for the lack of benefit from knowledge of prognosis is that most of the prognostic data is derived from studies that did not follow accepted principles for the conduct of prognostic studies. It is recommended that for biomarker prognostic studies the REMARK guidelines are followed or that studies satisfy the requirements outlined in the Quality in Prognosis Studies tool.[59,60] These are (1) prospective studies of patients investigated in a defined clinical setting for suspected or confirmed PE; (2) include patients consecutively in an unselected manner; (3) report on all-cause mortality, PE-related mortality, recurrent venous thromboembolism, major bleeding or intensive care unit admission, or on some composite of these 5 outcomes, so-called complicated clinical course, with a requirement for a priori, objective definitions; (4) used predefined time points for the outcome(s), ideally addressing early mortality risk; and (5) in the case of biomarkers describe the specific biomarker assays and use an a priori laboratory cutoff value for an abnormal result. Studies included in meta-analyses should be evaluated to have a low risk of bias across all domains of the Quality in Prognosis Studies tool. Unfortunately, to date no study have demonstrated an improvement in mortality rates after the implementation of a risk stratification strategy to guide treatment but it is important that work continue in this area. Research using management strategies or safer pharmacoinvasive treatments are ongoing (NCT02811237, NCT03988842, PEITHO-III study) **(Table 1)**.

DISCLOSURE

Dr P.S. Wells has received honoraria for Advisory Board meetings from Bayer Healthcare, Sanofi, and Daiichi Sankyo, and research funding from BMS/Pfizer.

REFERENCES

1. Gussoni G, Frasson S, Regina ML, et al. Three-month mortality rate and clinical predictors in patients with venous thromboembolism and cancer. Findings from the RIETE registry. Thromb Res 2013;131:24–30.
2. Ageno W, Mantovani LG, Haas S, et al. Safety and effectiveness of oral rivaroxaban versus standard anticoagulation for the treatment of symptomatic deep-vein thrombosis (XALIA): an international, prospective, non-interventional study. Lancet Haematol 2016;3:e12–21.
3. Kasper W, Konstantinides S, Geibel A, et al. Management strategies and determinants of outcome in acute major pulmonary embolism: results of a multicenter registry. J Am Coll Cardiol 1997;30:1165–71.
4. Keller K, Hobohm L, Ebner M, et al. Trends in thrombolytic treatment and outcomes of acute pulmonary embolism in Germany. Eur Heart J 2019. https://doi.org/10.1093/eurheartj/ehz236.
5. Quezada CA, Bikdeli B, Barrios D, et al. Meta-analysis of prevalence and short-term prognosis of hemodynamically unstable patients with symptomatic acute pulmonary embolism. Am J Cardiol 2019;123:684–9.
6. Barritt DW, Jordan SC. Anticoagulant drugs in the treatment of pulmonary embolism. A controlled trial. Lancet 1960;1:1309–12.
7. Heriot GS, Pitman AG, Gonzales M, et al. The four horsemen: clinicopathological correlation in 407 hospital autopsies. Intern Med J 2010;40:626–32.
8. Konstantinides SV, Torbicki A, Agnelli G, et al, Task Force for the Diagnosis and Management of Acute Pulmonary Embolism of the European Society of Cardiology (ESC). 2014 ESC guidelines on the diagnosis and management of acute pulmonary embolism. Eur Heart J 2014;35:3033–69, 3069a–3069k.
9. Kraaijpoel N, Tritschler T, Guillo E, et al. Definitions, adjudication, and reporting of pulmonary embolism-related death in clinical studies: a systematic review. J Thromb Haemost 2019. https://doi.org/10.1111/jth.14570.
10. Carson JL, Kelley MA, Duff A, et al. The clinical course of pulmonary embolism. N Engl J Med 1992;326:1240–5.
11. Girard P, Penaloza A, Parent F, et al. Reproducibility of clinical events adjudications in a trial of venous thromboembolism prevention. J Thromb Haemost 2017;15:662–9.
12. Roberts ISD, Benamore RE, Benbow EW, et al. Post-mortem imaging as an alternative to autopsy in the diagnosis of adult deaths: a validation study. Lancet 2012;379:136–42.

13. Kline JA, Hernandez-Nino J, Jones AE, et al. Prospective study of the clinical features and outcomes of emergency department patients with delayed diagnosis of pulmonary embolism. Acad Emerg Med 2007;14:592–8.

14. Torres-Macho J, Mancebo-Plaza AB, Crespo-Giménez A, et al. Clinical features of patients inappropriately undiagnosed of pulmonary embolism. Am J Emerg Med 2013;31:1646–50.

15. Goldhaber SZ, Visani L, De Rosa M. Acute pulmonary embolism: clinical outcomes in the international cooperative pulmonary embolism registry (ICOPER). Lancet 1999;353:1386–9.

16. Sweet PH, Armstrong T, Chen J, et al. Fatal pulmonary embolism update: 10 years of autopsy experience at an academic medical center. JRSM Short Rep 2013;4. 2042533313489824.

17. Meyer G, Collignon MA, Guinet F, et al. Comparison of perfusion lung scanning and angiography in the estimation of vascular obstruction in acute pulmonary embolism. Eur J Nucl Med 1990;17:315–9.

18. Qanadli SD, El Hajjam M, Vieillard-Baron A, et al. New CT index to quantify arterial obstruction in pulmonary embolism: comparison with angiographic index and echocardiography. AJR Am J Roentgenol 2001;176:1415–20.

19. Mastora I, Remy-Jardin M, Masson P, et al. Severity of acute pulmonary embolism: evaluation of a new spiral CT angiographic score in correlation with echocardiographic data. Eur Radiol 2003;13:29–35.

20. Vedovati MC, Germini F, Agnelli G, et al. Prognostic role of embolic burden assessed at computed tomography angiography in patients with acute pulmonary embolism: systematic review and meta-analysis. J Thromb Haemost 2013;11:2092–102.

21. Alkinj B, Pannu BS, Apala DR, et al. Saddle vs nonsaddle pulmonary embolism: clinical presentation, hemodynamics, management, and outcomes. Mayo Clin Proc 2017;92:1511–8.

22. Gandara E, Bose G, Erkens P, et al. Outcomes of saddle pulmonary embolism: a nested case-control study: letters to the editor. J Thromb Haemost 2011;9:867–9.

23. Barrios D, Rosa-Salazar V, Morillo R, et al. Prognostic significance of right heart thrombi in patients with acute symptomatic pulmonary embolism. Chest 2017;151:409–16.

24. Barrios D, Chavant J, Jiménez D, et al. Treatment of right heart thrombi associated with acute pulmonary embolism. Am J Med 2017;130:588–95.

25. Becattini C, Cohen AT, Agnelli G, et al. Risk stratification of patients with acute symptomatic pulmonary embolism based on presence or absence of lower extremity DVT. Chest 2016;149:192–200.

26. Mismetti P, Laporte S, Pellerin O, et al. Effect of a retrievable inferior vena cava filter plus anticoagulation vs anticoagulation alone on risk of recurrent pulmonary embolism: a randomized clinical trial. JAMA 2015;313:1627.

27. Hochuli M, Duewell S, Frauchiger B. Quantitative d-dimer levels and the extent of venous thromboembolism in CT angiography and lower limb ultrasonography. Vasa 2007;36:267–74.

28. Rydman R, Söderberg M, Larsen F, et al. d-Dimer and simplified pulmonary embolism severity index in relation to right ventricular function. Am J Emerg Med 2013;31:482–6.

29. Keller K, Beule J, Schulz A, et al. D-dimer for risk stratification in haemodynamically stable patients with acute pulmonary embolism. Adv Med Sci 2015;60:204–10.

30. Becattini C, Lignani A, Masotti L, et al. D-dimer for risk stratification in patients with acute pulmonary embolism. J Thromb Thrombolysis 2012;33:48–57.
31. Barco S, Ende-Verhaar YM, Becattini C, et al. Differential impact of syncope on the prognosis of patients with acute pulmonary embolism: a systematic review and meta-analysis. Eur Heart J 2018;39:4186–95.
32. Conget F, Otero R, Jiménez D, et al. Short-term clinical outcome after acute symptomatic pulmonary embolism. Thromb Haemost 2008;100:937–42.
33. Kearon C, Akl EA, Comerota AJ, et al. Antithrombotic therapy for VTE disease. Chest 2012;141:e419S–96S.
34. Wan S, Quinlan DJ, Agnelli G, et al. Thrombolysis compared with heparin for the initial treatment of pulmonary embolism: a meta-analysis of the randomized controlled trials. Circulation 2004;110:744–9.
35. Kabrhel C, Van Hylckama Vlieg A, Muzikanski A, et al. Multicenter evaluation of the YEARS criteria in emergency department patients evaluated for pulmonary embolism. Acad Emerg Med 2018;25:987–94.
36. Donzé J, Le Gal G, Fine MJ, et al. Prospective validation of the pulmonary embolism severity index. a clinical prognostic model for pulmonary embolism. Thromb Haemost 2008;100:943–8.
37. Zhou X-Y, Ben S-Q, Chen H-L, et al. The prognostic value of pulmonary embolism severity index in acute pulmonary embolism: a meta-analysis. Respir Res 2012; 13:111.
38. Vanni S, Nazerian P, Pepe G, et al. Comparison of two prognostic models for acute pulmonary embolism: clinical vs. right ventricular dysfunction-guided approach. J Thromb Haemost 2011;9:1916–23.
39. Zondag W, den Exter PL, Crobach MJT, et al. Comparison of two methods for selection of out of hospital treatment in patients with acute pulmonary embolism. Thromb Haemost 2013;109:47–52.
40. Wicki J, Perneger TV, Junod AF, et al. Assessing clinical probability of pulmonary embolism in the emergency ward: a simple score. Arch Intern Med 2001; 161:92–7.
41. Kavasoglu ME, Eken C, Eray O, et al. Value of high-sensitive cardiac troponin in predicting mortality in the emergency department. Clin Lab 2016;62:1483 9.
42. Eggers KM, Jernberg T, Lindahl B. Cardiac troponin elevation in patients without a specific diagnosis. J Am Coll Cardiol 2019;73:1–9.
43. Weekes AJ, Thacker G, Troha D, et al. Diagnostic accuracy of right ventricular dysfunction markers in normotensive emergency department patients with acute pulmonary embolism. Ann Emerg Med 2016;68:277–91.
44. Barco S, Mahmoudpour SH, Planquette B, et al. Prognostic value of right ventricular dysfunction or elevated cardiac biomarkers in patients with low-risk pulmonary embolism: a systematic review and meta-analysis. Eur Heart J 2019;40: 902–10.
45. Waxman DA, Hecht S, Schappert J, et al. A model for troponin i as a quantitative predictor of in-hospital mortality. J Am Coll Cardiol 2006;48:1755–62.
46. Bajaj A, Rathor P, Sehgal V, et al. Risk stratification in acute pulmonary embolism with heart-type fatty acid-binding protein: a meta-analysis. J Crit Care 2015;30: 1151.e1–7.
47. Bajaj A, Rathor P, Sehgal V, et al. Prognostic value of biomarkers in acute non-massive pulmonary embolism: a systematic review and meta-analysis. Lung 2015;193:639–51.
48. Daniel KR, Courtney DM, Kline JA. Assessment of cardiac stress from massive pulmonary embolism with 12-Lead ECG. Chest 2001;120:474–81.

49. Shopp JD, Stewart LK, Emmett TW, et al. Findings from 12-lead electrocardiography that predict circulatory shock from pulmonary embolism: systematic review and meta-analysis. Acad Emerg Med 2015;22:1127–37.
50. Grifoni S, Olivotto I, Cecchini P, et al. Short-term clinical outcome of patients with acute pulmonary embolism, normal blood pressure, and echocardiographic right ventricular dysfunction. Circulation 2000;101:2817–22.
51. Wolfe MW, Lee RT, Feldstein ML, et al. Prognostic significance of right ventricular hypokinesis and perfusion lung scan defects in pulmonary embolism. Am Heart J 1994;127:1371–5.
52. Kreit JW. The impact of right ventricular dysfunction on the prognosis and therapy of normotensive patients with pulmonary embolism. Chest 2004;125:1539–45.
53. Cho JH, Sridharan GK, Kim SH, et al. Right ventricular dysfunction as an echocardiographic prognostic factor in hemodynamically stable patients with acute pulmonary embolism: a meta-analysis. BMC Cardiovasc Disord 2014;14:64.
54. Meinel FG, Nance JW, Schoepf UJ, et al. Predictive value of computed tomography in acute pulmonary embolism: systematic review and meta-analysis. Am J Med 2015;128:747–59.e2.
55. Hobohm L, Hellenkamp K, Hasenfuß G, et al. Comparison of risk assessment strategies for not-high-risk pulmonary embolism. Eur Respir J 2016;47:1170–8.
56. Bova C, Sanchez O, Prandoni P, et al. Identification of intermediate-risk patients with acute symptomatic pulmonary embolism. Eur Respir J 2014;44:694–703.
57. Jimenez D, Lobo JL, Fernandez-Golfin C, et al. Effectiveness of prognosticating pulmonary embolism using the ESC algorithm and the Bova score. Thromb Haemost 2016;115:827–34.
58. Meyer G, Vicaut E, Danays T, et al. Fibrinolysis for patients with intermediate-risk pulmonary embolism. N Engl J Med 2014;370:1402–11.
59. McShane LM, Altman DG, Sauerbrei W, et al. REporting recommendations for tumour MARKer prognostic studies (REMARK). Br J Cancer 2005;93:387–91.
60. Hayden JA, van der Windt DA, Cartwright JL, et al. Assessing bias in studies of prognostic factors. Ann Intern Med 2013;158:280–6.

Overview of Management of Intermediate- and High-Risk Pulmonary Embolism

Victor F. Tapson, MD[a],*, Aaron S. Weinberg, MD, MPhil[b]

KEYWORDS

- Intermediate-risk • Submassive pulmonary embolism • High-risk
- Massive pulmonary embolism • Anticoagulation • Thrombolysis
- Catheter-directed therapy • Simplified pulmonary embolism severity index

KEY POINTS

- Anticoagulation should be initiated as soon as possible when pulmonary embolism (PE) is strongly suspected, if the risk of bleeding is deemed acceptable.
- Risk stratification should be considered when PE is suspected and a plan finalized once the diagnosis is confirmed.
- Therapy more aggressive than anticoagulation should be strongly considered in high-risk (massive) PE.
- Intermediate-risk PE is subdivided into intermediate-low and intermediate-high-risk groups; anticoagulation is generally appropriate for the former.
- Intermediate-high-risk PE is a heterogeneous category; a careful assessment of patient appearance, vital signs, oxygenation, echocardiographic parameters, right ventricular biomarkers, clot burden, and comorbidities should be undertaken to aid in therapeutic decisions.

INTRODUCTION

The goal of this article is to first define high-risk (massive) pulmonary embolism (PE) and intermediate-risk (submassive) PE and then to review the overall management strategies of these entities. Because risk stratification is intimately tied to PE management, the authors offer a brief overview of this concept. Other sections in this issue offer more detailed descriptions of risk-stratification approaches and specific management strategies, including systemic thrombolysis, catheter-directed strategies,

Funding: Research grants (paid to institution) - Bayer, BMS, Daiichi, Inari, Janssen, Penumbra. Advisory boards / consulting - Bayer, BMS, Inari, Janssen, Penumbra, Thrombolex.
[a] Pulmonary and Critical Care Medicine, Cedars-Sinai Medical Center, Thalians Building Room w155, 8730 Alden Drive, Los Angeles, CA 90048, USA; [b] Cedars-Sinai Medical Center, Thalians Building, 8730 Alden Drive, Los Angeles, CA 90048, USA
* Corresponding author.
E-mail address: victor.tapson@cshs.org

and surgical embolectomy, as well as extracorporeal membrane oxygenation (ECMO); the authors offer an overview but leave details of the precise strategies to the other respective article authors.

DEFINITIONS

The terms "high risk" and "intermediate risk" have been gradually replacing "massive PE" and "submassive PE," respectively, in the modern PE literature and guidelines, and although they remain interchangeable, the division of intermediate risk into intermediate-low- and intermediate-high-risk PE has made this particular term more useful.[1] Furthermore, some clinicians, including radiologists, have continued to erroneously use the terms "submassive" and "massive" to refer to the actual clot burden on imaging; these terms should be used as defined above. The authors use the newer nomenclature. Importantly, high-risk, intermediate-risk, and low-risk PE all represent heterogeneous categories.

High-Risk (Massive) Pulmonary Embolism

Historically, the definition of massive PE has evolved. The definition used for a large thrombolytic therapy trial in acute PE several decades ago required a baseline Miller angiographic score of at least 17/34 and mean pulmonary artery pressure of ≥ 20 mm Hg.[2] In recent years, the definition of high-risk/massive acute PE has not included any specific anatomic clot burden requirement but simply refers to those emboli causing hemodynamic instability. Although high-risk PE can itself be stratified (**Box 1**), there are no clear evidence-based treatment recommendations that distinguish these scenarios. The term "high-risk PE" implies that therapy more aggressive than anticoagulation should be strongly considered.

High-risk, intermediate-risk, and low-risk PE all represent heterogeneous categories. For example, a patient with high-risk PE may have suffered a pulseless with electrical activity (PEA) arrest and be requiring very high-dose vasopressor support

---

Box 1
Categories of high-risk (massive) pulmonary embolism

Supermassive/catastrophic PE
- Cardiac arrest/need for cardiopulmonary resuscitation[a]
- Obstructive shock: Hypotension requiring pressor therapy with evidence of end-organ hypoperfusion (AMS, cold/clammy, oliguria, elevated lactate) but not resulting in cardiac arrest[a]

Systemic hypotension: Systolic blood pressure (BP) <90 mm Hg or systolic BP drop ≥ 40 mm Hg, lasting longer than 15 minutes, caused by pulmonary artery obstruction, but requiring only low-dose, or no vasopressor therapy[b]

Severe hypoxemia/acute respiratory failure[c]

[a] Cardiac arrest is most commonly pulseless with electrical activity. Patients with PE and underlying comorbid disease (eg, sepsis, left ventricular dysfunction, severe pneumonia, or other cardiopulmonary disease) may meet criteria for high-risk PE based on these hemodynamic criteria with a less extensive clot burden.

[b] Patients may deteriorate from low- or intermediate-risk PE, or from a less severely ill high-risk PE scenario, transitioning to a more critically ill status because of recurrent PE and/or worsening right ventricular dysfunction. Trends are important to closely observe.

[c] When very high O_2 requirements or requirement for mechanical ventilation results from acute PE, generally other features, such as severe right ventricular failure and hypotension, are also present.

or ECMO, or could be awake, alert, and simply have a systolic blood pressure (BP) <90 mm Hg for more than 15 minutes, or a systolic BP drop from 140 mm Hg to 95 mm Hg (ie, >40 mm Hg drop). The clinical approach may differ.

Intermediate-Risk Pulmonary Embolism

Intermediate-risk PE has been more variably defined than high-risk PE and has historically implied right ventricular (RV) dysfunction in the absence of hypotension. These patients were described as the "middle group" several decades ago and were the patients who generated the most controversy over whether thrombolysis should be administered.[3] More specifically, this middle group was defined by some investigators as patients with acute PE with evidence of RV abnormalities defined in several different ways, including elevated pulmonary artery pressure, RV dilation (RV appearing larger than the left ventricle on apical or subcostal view), paradoxic septal wall motion, loss of inspiratory collapse of the inferior vena cava, or tricuspid regurgitation.[4] Sanchez and colleagues[5] performed a (selective) metaanalysis and calculated an odds ratio for short-term mortality for RV dysfunction on echocardiography (defined variably) of 2.53 (95% confidence interval 1.17–5.50). RV dysfunction can vary from very mild to very severe; acute PE associated with very mild RV dysfunction in the absence of recurrent PE, for example, would appear very unlikely to result in an adverse outcome. These earlier definitions did not include cardiac biomarkers or clinical criteria, and although perhaps practical at the time, the definition has evolved.

Computed tomographic (CT) scan measurements of RV dilation also appear to be accurate and reproducible even when radiology residents are performing the measurement.[6] These measurements have been shown to predict adverse short-term events, including in-hospital death, 30-day mortality, and mortality at 3 months; RV diameter divided by left ventricular (LV) diameter greater than 0.9 (4-chamber view) has been a commonly used definition in clinical trials.[7] Other metaanalytic data using a CTA RV/LV ratio of 0.9 or 1.0 also support this poor outcome.[8] RV/LV ratio by computed tomographic angiography (CTA) as a measure of RV dysfunction has been shown to correlate well with echocardiographic parameters.[9–11] Because many studies have used a very mild increase in RV/LV (eg, 0.9 as lower limit) for inclusion,[7,8] many *mildly* abnormal cases have been included. Thus, it is difficult to use this specific cutoff value as a decision point for more aggressive therapy in clinical practice.

Biomarkers, including troponin and brain natriuretic peptide (BNP)/NT-pro BNP, have proven to be effective predictors of outcome in acute PE with metaanalyses supporting this finding for both troponin[12] and BNP/NT-pro BNP.[13] These biomarkers have been included more recently in the definition of intermediate-risk PE, although the most recent European Society of Cardiology (ESC) guidelines have focused on troponin, noting that these other biomarkers may also be useful (1 ESC 2019). It should be emphasized that elevations of either or both of these biomarkers, *independent of other parameters of severity*, should not be used to make clinical decisions. Notably, D-dimer testing has been shown to not only be useful in ruling out the clinical diagnosis of acute PE but also in predicting severity.[14] Finally, other prognostic biomarker measurements have been studied and may be useful, including heart-type fatty acid–binding protein, although this is not currently widely available.[15]

The pulmonary embolism severity index

Over time, the definition of submassive/intermediate-risk PE evolved to include specific clinical criteria.[16] Of the clinical criteria, the Pulmonary Embolism Severity Index (PESI) and simplified Pulmonary Embolism Severity Index (sPESI) have both been validated for predicting 30-day mortality in patients with acute PE.[17–20]

The sPESI uses 6 risk factors (as compared with 11 risk factors in the original PESI score).[18,19] An sPESI score of 0 predicts a short-term mortality risk of 2.5% and a negative predictive value of 97.5% compared with the original PESI. A metaanalysis of 21 studies that included an aggregate of 50,000 patients demonstrated that both PESI and sPESI are equally effective in identifying patients with *low-risk* PE.[21] Because the sPESI serves the same purpose as PESI but is much simpler, the authors prefer it and do not calculate the PESI routinely; sPESI is quite simple for any clinician to memorize and use.

In 2014, ESC guidelines incorporated the PESI/sPESI into the definition of intermediate-risk PE in order to integrate clinical status and comorbidities.[16] Intermediate-risk PE was defined as a patient with PESI III–IV (or sPESI ≥1), *or* RV dysfunction based on either echocardiography *or* an elevated troponin. Furthermore, the intermediate-risk category has been subdivided into intermediate low risk and intermediate high risk. Intermediate-low-risk acute PE is defined a PESI III–IV or sPESI score greater than 0, or RV dysfunction by *either* echocardiography *or* an abnormal troponin, whereas intermediate-high-risk acute PE is defined as RV dysfunction by *both* echocardiography *and* an abnormal troponin, with or without an abnormal PESI or sPESI. It should be emphasized that a patient is still designated intermediate risk if RV dysfunction is present even if the sPESI is zero (**Box 2, Table 1**).

It should be noted that other scoring systems have been studied for risk stratification of acute PE; these are discussed in another article in this issue. The authors have focused on sPESI based on its incorporation into the definition of intermediate-risk PE.

Several clinical criteria appear to be helpful in the risk-stratification process and can serve as predictors of mortality in acute PE; thus, they are commonly included when assessing the PE patient. These criteria include clinical appearance, respiratory rate, pulmonary embolic burden,[22,23] D-dimer level[14] (ie, *severity* of the elevation in D-dimer), and residual deep vein thrombosis (DVT).[24] Residual DVT in the setting of acute PE has been shown to be associated with a 2-fold increase in mortality.[24] However, clear changes in the PE treatment plan cannot generally be recommended based on residual DVT in the absence of severe acute DVT symptoms or phlegmasia.

Box 2
Intermediate-risk pulmonary embolism

Hemodynamically stable[a]

Each of the following 3 conditions (alone) defines intermediate-risk PE:
- sPESI >0 (or PESI III–IV) alone = intermediate-risk PE
- RV dysfunction alone = intermediate-risk PE[b]
- Troponin elevation alone = intermediate-risk PE[b]

Intermediate-low risk = RV dysfunction[c] *or* elevated troponin

Intermediate-high risk = RV dysfunction[c] *and* elevated troponin

[a] This implies no cardiac arrest or hypotension (systolic blood pressure not dropping below 90 mm Hg for ≥15 minutes because of PE, no need for vasopressors, and systolic blood pressure has not dropped by >40 mm Hg compared with baseline).
[b] Signs of RV dysfunction by echocardiography (or CTA) or elevated cardiac biomarker levels may be present, despite a calculated PESI of I–II or an sPESI of 0; these patients are still classified as intermediate risk.
[c] RV dysfunction is generally defined by depressed RV function by echocardiography but a significantly dilated right ventricle by chest CTA also suggests RV dysfunction. There is not a specific echocardiographic parameter, which identifies an intermediate-risk patient; several clinical trials have used RV/LV >0.9 or 1.0 to designate an abnormal right ventricle (see text).

Table 1	
The simplified pulmonary embolism severity index[a]	
Criterion	**Points**
Age >80 y	1
History of cancer	1
History of chronic lung disease	1
History of heart failure	1
Heart rate >110 beats/min	1
Systolic blood pressure <100 mm Hg	1
Oxygen saturation <90%	1

[a] A low-risk sPESI (score of 0) predicts a short-term mortality risk of 2.5% and a negative predictive value of 97.5% comparable to the original PESI score.

Although the aforementioned parameters are very useful clinically, many have not been incorporated into formal risk-stratification recommendations (**Box 3**).

Whether clot burden measured by CTA predicts adverse prognosis has been controversial in studies published to date, probably because of differences in the populations studied in terms of severity of PE; several studies suggest that it does.[23] Logic dictates that the larger the PE, the more likely an adverse outcome. For example, PE that is so extensive that it causes near complete pulmonary arterial obstruction is likely to be associated with a higher risk of RV failure and death. Nonetheless, patients with very extensive PE may be quite clinically stable so that clot burden *alone* should not be used to make therapeutic decisions. Clot burden has not found its way into the intermediate- or high-risk definitions.

Box 3
Clinical parameters to consider in acute intermediate-risk pulmonary embolism

Appearance

Respiratory rate

Heart rate

Blood pressure

Clot burden by CTA or VQ scan

RV function by echocardiogram

Troponin

BNP/NT-pro BNP

Oxygen requirement

Lactate

Residual DVT

Although there are cutoff values for some of these parameters, defining, for example, an abnormal sPESI, such values do not necessarily guide clinical decisions. For example, the heart rate criterion for sPESI is >110/min, but a heart rate of 110/min does not necessarily mandate more aggressive therapy than anticoagulation. A heart rate of 130/min would appear more likely to be associated with a higher mortality and influence clinicians to be more aggressive, but there are no data proving that such an approach would reduce mortality. Clinicians should consider all of these parameters, use clinical gestalt as well as any apparent trends, and plan the therapeutic approach.

POTENTIAL BENEFITS OF ACUTE PULMONARY EMBOLISM THERAPY

Anticoagulation has proven to improve mortality in acute PE.[25] It has been generally accepted that acute high-risk PE is a high-mortality entity and that more aggressive therapy than anticoagulation is indicated. However, although intermediate-high risk PE appears to have a higher mortality than intermediate-low risk PE,[20,21] there has been no proven mortality benefit by increasing the level of aggressiveness of therapy in the intermediate-high risk group. Furthermore, it remains unclear whether early reperfusion treatment, for example, thrombolysis, has an impact on clinical symptoms, functional limitation, or the development of pulmonary hypertension.

ACUTE PULMONARY EMBOLISM: SUPPORTIVE THERAPY AND GENERAL CONCEPTS

Treatment of acute PE is not black and white and depends on the severity of the clinical parameters, the perceived bleeding risk, and the therapeutic options available to the team of physicians treating the patient.

The Pulmonary Embolism Response Team

The authors believe the pulmonary embolism response team (PERT) concept facilitates the care of high- and intermediate-risk patients as well as other complex venous thromboembolism scenarios.[26] This concept has evolved based on the lack of a strong evidence base directing clinicians in these settings. Rapidly implementing a team of clinicians well versed in PE to assist the emergency department or primary team caring for an intermediate- or high-risk PE patient can expedite sound clinical decisions.[26] Furthermore, an expert multidisciplinary team can offer recommendations in many other clinical scenarios, such as heparin-induced thrombocytopenia, high bleeding risk, symptomatic extensive DVT, complex surgical or comorbid settings, and many other situations. These multidisciplinary teams often include specialists in pulmonary/critical care, cardiology, hospital medicine, interventional radiology, hematology, clinical pharmacy, vascular medicine, vascular surgery, and cardiothoracic surgery.[27] Naturally, when relevant, other specialists, such as neurosurgery or obstetrics/gynecology, become involved. The PERT concept is evolving, and the PERT Consortium, a 501(c)3 nonprofit organization, sponsors an annual multidisciplinary PE symposium. Clinical guidelines for PE management have been published by the PERT Consortium.[28] The management of intermediate- and high-risk PE needs continued research, and the PERT Consortium encourages this and offers multidisciplinary expert input in the meantime.[28] Importantly, retrospective studies examining PERT programs and outcomes have found that most patients evaluated by PERTs are treated with anticoagulation and not more invasive techniques.[26]

Anticoagulation

Importantly, anticoagulation should be initiated immediately upon diagnosing acute PE or when there is a high or intermediate probability of PE as the workup is in progress, unless the bleeding risk appears high; this is a grade 1C recommendation in 2019 ESC/European Respiratory Society guidelines.[1]

There are no clear guidelines on which anticoagulant is appropriate to initiate in intermediate- and high-risk patients. The markedly hypotensive high-risk patient who is perfusing very poorly may be best served by a direct intravenous (IV) approach, that is, unfractionated heparin rather than subcutaneous low-molecular-weight heparin (LMWH). Most other patients are probably good candidates for initial LMWH based on its superior bioavailability and lack of need for monitoring in most cases. After the initial dose, the clinician can focus on other aspects of care rather than being preoccupied with whether a therapeutic level has been achieved. The clinicians involved in caring for these patients should have a good understanding of their potential interventionalist's preferences. For example, although most interventionalists are comfortable proceeding with a catheter-directed thrombolysis procedure, extraction technique, or inferior vena cava (IVC) filter after LMWH administration, some might prefer the shorter-acting IV standard heparin in such cases. The authors' belief is that most patients should be administered LMWH regardless of whether a procedure is planned based on the above rationale. When the patient (with or without an interventional technique) is deemed clinically stable and has been observed long enough without deterioration (generally at 24–48 hours), transition to oral anticoagulation is appropriate. Most commonly, this would be a direct oral anticoagulant unless contraindicated. Notably, in the large randomized PEITHO trial, the mean time between randomization and death or hemodynamic deterioration was 1.79 ± 1.6 days in the heparin-only arm.[29]

Any PE patient who cannot be anticoagulated should undergo IVC filter placement. If no residual DVT is present, a delay in placement may be acceptable; there is no standard of care for how soon a filter must be placed. However, a patient who has just suffered acute PE is likely to be at continued risk and could form new DVT and reembolize.

Oxygen and mechanical ventilation
Oxygen therapy should be initiated unless a patient has a normal O_2 saturation and is comfortable at rest and with at least minimal ambulation. Oxygen saturation may be deceptive; a saturation measure, for example, of 98% does not guarantee normal gas exchange. The alveolar-arterial difference may be quite abnormal in such a patient who is breathing hard and driving down the P_{CO_2} to compensate. When necessary, noninvasive ventilation or oxygenation through a high-flow nasal cannula is favored over intubation, but the latter is sometimes unavoidable.

Naturally, when a patient with impending respiratory failure requires intubation, it should be done cautiously, realizing that positive pressure may adversely affect a failing right ventricle.[30] Intubation should be performed by an experienced anesthesiologist; a cardiac anesthesiologist is ideal when available. Mild to moderate hemodynamic instability, including pressor-dependent hypotension, does not automatically imply the need for intubation: an awake patient may improve significantly when pressors are added.

When mechanical ventilation is required, tidal volumes in the range of 6 mL/kg lean body weight should be used, and minimal positive end-expiratory pressure should be applied to keep the end-inspiratory plateau pressure less than 30 cm H_2O. If intubation is needed, anesthetic drugs less prone to cause hypotension should be used; an induction agent such as etomidate (0.2–0.4 mg/kg) is hemodynamically neutral and may help to limit hypotension; midazolam, for example, is more likely to cause hypotension.[31] Ketamine is also an alternative agent that offers hemodynamic benefit; a randomized trial is currently comparing the hemodynamic effects of etomidate and ketamine during rapid sequence intubation.[32]

Fluid administration and vasoactive therapy
No clear guidelines exist for fluid administration in the hemodynamically unstable PE patient. If the central venous pressure appears to be low, a cautious fluid challenge (eg, ≤500 mL) can be undertaken; this may increase the cardiac index in patients with acute PE.[33] However, overaggressive fluid administration may overload the right ventricle, leading to a reduction in cardiac output.[33,34] Assessment of central venous

pressure by echocardiographic imaging of the IVC can be useful (a small/collapsible IVC in the setting of acute high-risk PE strongly suggests hypovolemia). If the central venous pressure appears elevated, volume loading can be halted.

Use of vasopressors is based on hypotension together with evidence of underperfusion, for example, including a cold, clammy appearance and elevated lactate.

Norepinephrine, epinephrine, and high-dose dopamine have demonstrated favorable hemodynamic effects in acute PE with circulatory failure.[35,36] The authors rarely use dopamine based on its potential arrhythmogenic effects. Norepinephrine is a potent α1-adrenergic receptor agonist with modest β1-agonist activity, which renders it a powerful vasoconstrictor with less potent direct inotropic properties. It is probably the most commonly used vasopressor for acute PE.[35,36] Norepinephrine may be the preferred initial agent because α-mediated vasoconstriction leads to increased mean arterial pressure; also, its β1-mediated inotropic effect may improve RV function. Vasopressin can be added if norepinephrine doses are escalating in hopes of minimizing the increase in pulmonary vascular resistance.

Based on the results of a small series, the use of dobutamine has been considered in PE in the setting of a low cardiac index and normal BP. Although the use of this "inodilator" would appear logical for the failing right ventricle, in fact, raising the cardiac index may worsen ventilation/perfusion mismatch by redistributing flow to less obstructed vessels.[37] Furthermore, the thin-walled failing right ventricle may simply not respond to inotropic encouragement; thus, it is difficult to conceive how novel vasoactive agents could offer substantial benefit over available agents. Relieving obstruction or bypassing is crucial in patients with high-risk PE. In general, if dobutamine is used, the authors would use it concomitantly with another vasopressor. Circulatory support in high-risk acute PE is detailed in separate articles.

Intensive Care Unit Admission?

There are no clear guidelines regarding the need for intensive care unit (ICU) admission in acute PE. Patients with high-risk PE should be admitted to the ICU. Patients with intermediate-risk PE should be individualized. Patients with borderline hypotension, excessive tachypnea, and/or tachycardia (eg, heart rate >110/min), and those requiring more than low-flow O_2, should be considered for ICU admission. Patients who will receive or have already received thrombolysis should be admitted to the ICU when possible for closer monitoring, including careful observation for neurologic changes and bleeding. Hospitals vary, and the availability of monitoring, telemetry, and nighttime staff should be considered, and very importantly, clinical trends should be carefully scrutinized.

Anticoagulated patients, and in particular, those undergoing thrombolysis should be monitored for bleeding, as well as for heparin-induced thrombocytopenia. General symptom and neurologic assessment as well as vital signs and physical examinations should be carefully followed and may help identify bleeding and its potential source. Daily complete blood counts (for hemoglobin and platelets) are performed in hospitalized patients.

TREATMENT OF HIGH-RISK PULMONARY EMBOLISM

As described, this group is heterogeneous, and the treatment approaches depend on the available evidence and on the specific clinical circumstances. All patients require anticoagulation unless contraindicated. Even this is not always clear; a brain bleed 1 day before is different than spinal surgery 1 week before, and in turn, different than gastrointestinal bleeding episode 3 weeks before. Appropriate consultants should team up with regard to the risk of anticoagulation when the risk of bleeding is concerning. The general approach to high-risk PE is suggested in **Fig. 1**.

Catastrophic or Supermassive Pulmonary Embolism

The extreme scenario of proven acute PE causing cardiac arrest requiring advanced cardiac life support measures with cardiopulmonary resuscitation (CPR) and other aggressive supportive measures is often deemed "supermassive" or "catastrophic" PE. Systemic thrombolysis, surgical embolectomy, and ECMO are considered in such patients; occasionally, centers with rapidly responding clinicians (or PERTs) can successfully use catheter-directed approaches as well. Thrombolysis in the setting of CPR is not contraindicated, but resulting rib fractures with bleeding, pneumothorax, and cardiac tamponade may be worsened by thrombolysis. Unfortunately,

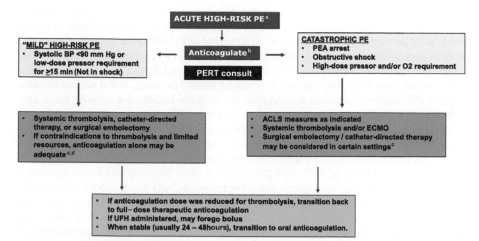

Fig. 1. High-risk acute PE: initial management. Anticoagulation should be initiated as soon as possible. When contraindicated, an IVC filter should be placed. Timing of filter depends on urgency of other interventions and may be done in conjunction with these. If the patient is too unstable to move, a bedside IVC filter may be placed. [a] The minimum requirement to meet the definition of high-risk PE is systolic BP <90 mm Hg for ≥15 minutes. However, high-risk PE is heterogeneous, ranging from the latter to catastrophic PE with cardiovascular collapse and PEA arrest. Management and use of specific therapies may vary based on the severity of the high-risk PE and on available resources. [b] IV heparin or LMWH. LMWH administration is not a contraindication to thrombolysis. Standard UFH is often used in anticipation of thrombolysis based on its shorter half-life. [c] Specific measures depend on details of the case and resources available. Contraindications to thrombolysis should be carefully considered. Systemic thrombolysis may be given at full dose or half dose; no clear guidelines differentiate the indications for the 2 dosing strategies. Relative contraindications, age, and body weight may aid in this decision. Catheter-directed therapy may use thrombolysis, or not. When thrombolysis is contraindicated, then a nonthrombolytic procedure should be used. There is no proven advantage of measuring fibrinogen levels for the purpose of guiding thrombolytic dose. Before and during systemic thrombolytic infusion, the heparin infusion may be stopped or reduced substantially. After thrombolysis, heparin may be reinitiated several hours later without a bolus. [d] If resources are limited and thrombolysis contraindicated, "mild" high-risk PE may sometimes be closely observed in the ICU with anticoagulation and supportive therapy, particularly if trends suggest improvement. Few outcome data exist on safety of transfer to tertiary care center. ACLS, advanced cardiac life support; CDT, catheter-directed therapy; UFH, unfractionated heparin.

the low cardiac output state during CPR is far from an ideal setting for thrombolytic penetration into the emboli.

If thrombolysis is administered in catastrophic PE, it is generally given by bolus or very rapidly. Systemic thrombolysis may be given at full dose or half dose; no clear guidelines differentiate the indications for the 2 dosing strategies. Relative and absolute contraindications should be considered, and age and body weight may aid in this decision; elderly patients are more likely to suffer intracranial hemorrhage and major bleeding.[29,38]

There is no proven advantage of measuring fibrinogen levels for the purpose of guiding thrombolytic dose. Before and during systemic thrombolytic infusion, the heparin infusion may be stopped or reduced substantially. In actuality, IV tissue type-plasminogen activator , the most commonly used thrombolytic agent, outlasts its apparent half-life because of thrombin-binding and the prolonged effects and longer half-life of its product, plasmin; however, the pharmacokinetics do not warrant prolonged avoidance of therapeutic anticoagulation when clinically indicated. In a clinical trial comparing thrombolysis followed by immediate heparin to heparin alone, only 1 intracranial hemorrhage was observed, in a patient who had sustained head trauma.[39] After thrombolysis, heparin is generally restarted within a few hours without a bolus.

Catheter-directed therapy may use thrombolysis, or not. When thrombolysis is contraindicated, then a nonthrombolytic procedure should be used. In the setting of catastrophic PE, catheter-directed approaches are feasible but require experience, a very well-organized team effort, and available resources. Although several catheter-based techniques have been used and are being studied, these techniques as well as systemic thrombolysis are reviewed in a separate article.

Patients with catastrophic PE with impending or actual PEA arrest are potential candidates for venoarterial ECMO. As ECMO teams have become more commonplace and response times and technology have improved, ECMO has become increasingly useful in these patients. In such patients, when ECMO is available, the decision must be made as to whether to administer bolus IV thrombolysis or whether to immediately cannulate for ECMO. Although immediate systemic thrombolysis has the potential to reverse hemodynamic compromise, the bleeding risk may complicate cannulation and successful ECMO. Surgical embolectomy combined with ECMO should be considered in critical patients with PE particularly with impending PEA arrest or after CPR has been initiated. These decisions cannot easily be standardized based on the few available pieces of outcome data and the individual variation in clinical specifics, resources and timing. The authors believe that PERTs facilitate these decisions.

Survival of critically ill patients on ECMO has been described in several case series,[40] but randomized controlled trials are exceedingly difficult to accomplish. ECMO is associated with a high incidence of complications, and patient selection and experience of the medical center are of critical importance. A critical evaluation of ECMO as well as other RV support methods is offered in separate articles.

High-Risk Pulmonary Embolism: The "More Stable" Patient

Although high-risk patients have increased mortality, some patients are less critically ill without the appearance of impending arrest. Based on the definition of high-risk PE, 1 end of the spectrum is the patient with a systolic BP of approximately 90 mm Hg requiring no pressors or perhaps low-dose norepinephrine (eg, 2–4 µg/min) who is awake and alert and, for example, slightly improved over the prior hour. Such patients are nearly always tachycardic and have severely abnormal RV function unless there is an additional contributor to the hypotension. These patients should be carefully risk assessed and individualized for systemic thrombolysis or catheter-directed therapy.

Although the evidence base for these therapies in such patients is weak, it is generally considered the standard of care to proceed with one of these interventions if available, in patients meeting the definition of high-risk PE if there are no contraindications, even if the patient is not requiring substantial hemodynamic support.[1]

TREATMENT OF INTERMEDIATE-RISK PULMONARY EMBOLISM

Anticoagulation is the cornerstone of PE therapy and is sufficient for low-risk as well as many intermediate-risk patients.[1,16] Those intermediate-risk patients with more advanced features or who are deteriorating can be considered for more advanced therapy. Those who deteriorate on or before anticoagulation and are now *high-risk* PE are treated as such. Those intermediate-risk patients who have not progressed to high-risk status, but have very concerning features, can be considered for therapeutic options, including catheter-directed clot extraction, and catheter-directed thrombolysis, although again, the evidence base for these approaches is weaker and such patients should be individualized. Recognizing the heterogeneity of these patients is important. For example, the intermediate-high-risk patient with sPESI greater than 0, a mildly abnormal right ventricle, and elevated troponin is not *automatically* a candidate for more advanced therapy than anticoagulation, despite that the data that this group *as a whole* have a higher risk of mortality at 30 days.

It is critical that the clinician recognize that each of the parameters that used to gauge severity should be closely scrutinized. Tachycardia might be a heart rate of 100/min or 130/min. RV dysfunction may be mild or very severe. A troponin elevation may be just above the upper limit of normal, or it may be hundreds of times that.

The authors' opinion is that the intermediate-low-risk patient (sPESI >0, who has either normal RV function and normal RV biomarkers, or mild RV dysfunction, *or* a mildly elevated troponin) should nearly always be managed with anticoagulation alone. The intermediate-high-risk, normotensive patient who appears comfortable on room air, with a heart rate of 112/min, for example, mildly depressed RV function, and a mildly elevated troponin would be a reasonable candidate for close observation in a monitored bed (or ICU) on anticoagulation because of the risk of early hemodynamic decompensation.[29] If symptoms and tachycardia, for example, worsen, ICU admission and more aggressive therapy should be considered. Depending on the precise conditions and resources, a catheter-directed approach might be considered for some intermediate-high-risk patients at some centers, although it should be recognized that although the RV/LV ratio has been shown to improve with such interventions, clinical outcomes, including mortality, have not been demonstrated to improve in these patients, perhaps in part because of inadequate trial sample size. The authors believe that well-designed clinical trials are essential in this area and that medical centers with the interest and capability should make every effort to participate.

Clinical trends may be critically important in decision making. Appearance, vital signs, and all parameters should be considered. Guidelines generally support aggressive therapy, such as systemic thrombolysis, in the intermediate-risk patient with clear signs of deterioration (American College of Chest Physicians).[41] Catheter-directed approaches may be considered, and their use depends on experience and the rapidity with which resources can be mobilized.[42] If, for any reason, anticoagulation has been discontinued at any point, it should be resumed as soon as deemed safe. The general therapeutic approach to intermediate-risk PE is shown in **Fig. 2**.

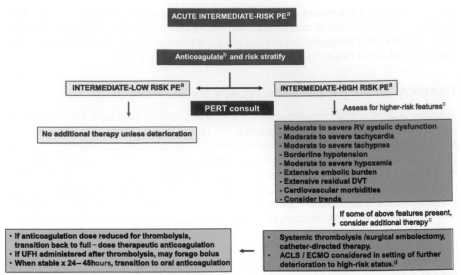

Fig. 2. Intermediate-risk acute PE: initial management. Intermediate-risk PE is a heterogeneous category with regard to severity. Anticoagulation should be initiated as soon as possible. When contraindicated, an IVC filter should be placed. [a] Intermediate-risk = sPESI greater than 0, and/or RV dysfunction and/or elevated troponin. Intermediate-low risk = any sPESI and RV dysfunction or elevated troponin. Intermediate-high-risk PE = any sPESI and RV dysfunction and elevated troponin. The definition of RV dysfunction varies and can be characterized echocardiographically based on RV wall motion, TAPSE, RV/LV ratio. Chest CTA can be used to indicate RV size, RV/LV ratio, furthermore, contrast reflux into the IVC/liver may indicate elevated PA pressure. Although intermediate-high-risk PE appears to have poorer outcomes than intermediate-low-risk PE, this distinction does not necessarily aid in treatment decisions. [b] IV heparin or LMWH unless contraindicated. [c] None of these higher-risk features clearly mandate more aggressive therapy but should be carefully taken into consideration. There is no particular number of, and no absolute cut-off values for, any of these measures that suggest the need for more aggressive therapy than anticoagulation. Use of a PERT with clinical expertise combined with gestalt, as well as clinical trends, should be considered. [d] Specific measures depend on details of the case and the resources available. Catheter-directed therapy may use thrombolysis, or not. When thrombolysis is deemed contraindicated, then a nonthrombolytic procedure should be used (see Fig. 1). CDT, catheter-directed therapy; PA, pulmonary arterial; TAPSE, tricuspid annular plane systolic excursion.

Finally, other clinical scenarios, such as clot-in-transit and paradoxic emboli, do not actually fit into the definitions of high-risk or intermediate-risk PE and are beyond the scope of this article but merit consideration.[43,44]

SUMMARY

Anticoagulation remains the best guarantee of reducing mortality in acute PE.[1,25,41] Patients with intermediate-risk (submassive) or high-risk (massive) PE have a higher mortality than low-risk patients. Patients with high-risk PE should be considered for more aggressive therapy. Both high- and intermediate-risk patients are heterogeneous, and this heterogeneity extends beyond the subdivision into intermediate-low and intermediate-high risk; more than simply categorizing a patient in this manner is required to guide therapy. Therapeutic approaches depend on a prompt, detailed evaluation of all parameters and on expertise that may be provided by multidisciplinary PERTs. More clinical trial data are needed to guide clinicians in the management of patients with acute intermediate- and high-risk PE.

DISCLOSURE

Authors have nothing to disclose.

REFERENCES

1. Konstantinides SV, Meyer G, Becattini C, et al. ESC guidelines for the diagnosis and management of acute pulmonary embolism developed in collaboration with the European Respiratory Society (ERS): the task force for the diagnosis and management of acute pulmonary embolism of the European Society of Cardiology (ESC). Eur Heart J 2019. https://doi.org/10.1093/eurheartj/ehz405.
2. Sors H, Pacouret G, Azarian R, et al. Hemodynamic effects of bolus vs 2-h infusion of alteplase in acute massive pulmonary embolism: a randomized controlled multicenter trial. Chest 1994;106:712–7.
3. Goldhaber SZ. Pulmonary embolism thrombolysis: broadening the paradigm for its administration. Circulation 1997;96:716–71.
4. Kasper W, Konstantinides S, Geibel A, et al. Management strategies and determinants of outcome in acute major pulmonary embolism: results of a multicenter registry. J Am Coll Cardiol 1997;30:1165–71.
5. Sanchez O, Trinquart L, Colombet I, et al. Prognostic value of right ventricular dysfunction in patients with haemodynamically stable pulmonary embolism: a systematic review. Eur Heart J 2008;29:1569–77.
6. Ende-Verhaar YM, Kroft LJM, Mos ICM, et al. Accuracy and reproducibility of CT right-to-left ventricular diameter measurement in patients with acute pulmonary embolism. PLoS One 2017;12:1–9.
7. Quiroz R, Kucher N, Schoepf UJ, et al. Right ventricular enlargement on chest computed tomography: prognostic role in acute pulmonary embolism. Circulation 2004;109:2401–4.
8. Becattini C, Agnelli G, Vedovati MC, et al. Multidetector computed tomography for acute pulmonary embolism: diagnosis and risk stratification in a single test. Eur Heart J 2011;32:1657–63.
9. Ozsu S, Karaman K, Mentese A, et al. Combined risk stratification with computed tomography/echocardiography and biomarkers in patients with normotensive pulmonary embolism. Thromb Res 2010;126:486–92.
10. Aribas A, Keskin S, Akilli H, et al. The use of axial diameters and CT obstruction scores for determining echocardiographic right ventricular dysfunction in patients with acute pulmonary embolism. Jpn J Radiol 2014;32:451–60.
11. Park JR, Chang SA, Jang SY, et al. Evaluation of right ventricular dysfunction and prediction of clinical outcomes in acute pulmonary embolism by chest computed tomography: comparisons with echocardiography. Int J Cardiovasc Imaging 2012;28:979–87.
12. Becattini C, Vedovati MC, Agnelli G. Prognostic value of troponins in acute pulmonary embolism: a meta-analysis. Circulation 2007;116:427–33.
13. Klok FA, Mos IC, Huisman MV. Brain-type natriuretic peptide levels in the prediction of adverse outcome in patients with pulmonary embolism: a systematic review and meta-analysis. Am J Respir Crit Care Med 2008;178:425–30.
14. Ghanima W, Abdelnoor M, Holmen LO, et al. D-dimer level is associated with the extent of pulmonary embolism. Thromb Res 2007;120:281–8.

15. Dellas C, Puls M, Lankeit M, et al. Elevated heart-type fatty acid-binding protein levels on admission predict an adverse outcome in normotensive patients with acute pulmonary embolism. J Am Coll Cardiol 2010;55:2150–7.
16. Konstantinides SV, Torbicki A, Agnelli G, et al. 2014 ESC guidelines on the diagnosis and management of acute pulmonary embolism: the task force for the diagnosis and management of acute pulmonary embolism of the European Society of Cardiology (ESC). Eur Heart J 2014;35:3033–80.
17. Donze J, Le Gal G, Fine MJ, et al. Prospective validation of the pulmonary embolism severity index. A clinical prognostic model for pulmonary embolism. Thromb Haemost 2008;100:943–8.
18. Aujesky D, Obrosky DS, Stone RA, et al. Derivation and validation of a prognostic model for pulmonary embolism. Am J Respir Crit Care Med 2005;172:1041–6.
19. Jimenez D, Aujesky D, Moores L, et al, RIETE Investigators. Simplification of the pulmonary embolism severity index for prognostication in patients with acute symptomatic pulmonary embolism. Arch Intern Med 2010;170:1383–9.
20. Righini M, Roy PM, Meyer G, et al. The simplified pulmonary embolism severity index (PESI): validation of a clinical prognostic model for pulmonary embolism. J Thromb Haemost 2011;9:2115–7.
21. Zhou XY, Ben SQ, Chen HL, et al. The prognostic value of pulmonary embolism severity index in acute pulmonary embolism: a meta-analysis. Respir Res 2012; 13:111.
22. Becattini C, Vedovati MC, Pruszczyk P, et al. Oxygen saturation or respiratory rate to improve risk stratification in hemodynamically stable patients with acute pulmonary embolism. J Thromb Haemost 2018;16:2397–402.
23. van der Meer RW, Pattynama PM, van Strijen MJ, et al. Right ventricular dysfunction and pulmonary obstruction index at helical CT: prediction of clinical outcome during 3-month follow-up in patients with acute pulmonary embolism. Radiology 2005;235:798–803.
24. Becatttini C, Cohen AT, Agnelli G, et al. Risk stratification of patients with acute symptomatic pulmonary embolism based on presence or absence of lower extremity DVT: systematic review and meta-analysis. Chest 2016;149:192–200.
25. Smith SB, Geske JB, Maguire JM, et al. Early anticoagulation is associated with reduced mortality for acute pulmonary embolism. Chest 2010;137:1382–90.
26. Kabrhel C, Rosovsky R, Channick R, et al. A multidisciplinary pulmonary response team: initial 30-month experience with a novel approach to delivery of care to patients with submassive and massive pulmonary embolism. Chest 2016;150:384–93.
27. Elbadawi A, Wright C, Patel D, et al. The impact of a multi-specialty team for high risk pulmonary embolism on resident and fellow education. Vasc Med 2018;23: 372–6.
28. Rivera-Lebron B, McDaniel M, Ahrar K, et al. Diagnosis, treatment and follow up of acute pulmonary embolism: consensus practice from the PERT Consortium. Clin Appl Thromb Hemost 2019;25:1–16.
29. Meyer G, Vicaut E, Danays T, et al, the PEITHO Investigators. Fibrinolysis for patients with intermediate-risk pulmonary embolism. N Engl J Med 2014;370: 1402–11.
30. Ventetuolo CE, Klinger JR. Management of acute right ventricular failure in the intensive care unit. Ann Am Thorac Soc 2014;11:811–22.
31. Choi YF, Wong TW, Lau CC. Midazolam is more likely to cause hypotension than etomidate in emergency department rapid sequence intubation. Emerg Med J 2004;21:700–2.

32. Evaluating the hemodynamic effects of ketamine versus etomidate during rapid sequence intubation. ClinicalTrials.gov Identifier NCT03545503.
33. Mercat A, Diehl JL, Meyer G, et al. Hemodynamic effects of fluid loading in acute massive pulmonary embolism. Crit Care Med 1999;27:540–4.
34. Ghignone M, Girling L, Prewitt RM. Volume expansion versus norepinephrine in treatment of a low cardiac output complicating an acute increase in right ventricular afterload in dogs. Anesthesiology 1984;60:132–5.
35. Layish DT, Tapson VF. Pharmacologic hemodynamic support in massive pulmonary embolism. Chest 1997;111:218–24.
36. Piazza G, Goldhaber SZ. The acutely decompensated right ventricle. Pathways for diagnosis and management. Chest 2005;128:1836–52.
37. Manier G, Castaing Y. Influence of cardiac output on oxygen exchange in acute pulmonary embolism. Am Rev Respir Dis 1992;145:130–6.
38. Chatterjee S, Chakraborty A, Weinberg I, et al. Thrombolysis for pulmonary embolism and risk of all-cause mortality, major bleeding, and intracranial hemorrhage: a meta-analysis. JAMA 2014;311:2414–21.
39. Goldhaber S, Come P, Lee R, et al. Alteplase versus heparin in acute pulmonary embolism: randomised trial assessing right-ventricular function and pulmonary perfusion. Lancet 1993;341(8844):507–11.
40. Corsi F, Lebreton G, Brechot N, et al. Life-threatening massive pulmonary embolism rescued by venoarterial-extracorporeal membrane oxygenation. Crit Care 2017;21:76.
41. Kearon CA, Akl EA, Ornelas J, et al. Antithrombotic therapy for VTE disease: CHEST guideline and expert panel report. Chest 2016;149:315–52.
42. Tapson VF, Jimenez D. Catheter-based approaches to acute pulmonary embolism. Semin Respir Crit Care Med 2017;38:73–83.
43. Patel M, Raza A, Murabia A, et al. Clot-in-transit: a therapeutic dilemma. Chest 2017;152:A1023.
44. Le Moigne E, Timsit S, Ben Salem D, et al. Patent foramen ovale and ischemic stroke in patients with pulmonary embolism: a prospective cohort study. Ann Intern Med 2019;170:756–63.

Thrombolysis in Pulmonary Embolism

An Evidence-Based Approach to Treating Life-Threatening Pulmonary Emboli

Eric Kaplovitch, MD, FRCPC[a],*, Joseph R. Shaw, MD[b],
James Douketis, MD, FRCPC[c]

KEYWORDS

- Thrombolysis • Pulmonary embolism • Massive • Submassive • Anticoagulation
- Venous thromboembolism

KEY POINTS

- Hemodynamically significant pulmonary embolism is associated with high morbidity and mortality, both via cardiorespiratory decompensation and the bleeding complications of treatment.
- Thrombolysis should be performed in patients with acute pulmonary embolism and evidence of systemic arterial hypotension ("massive PE") unless severe contraindications are present.
- Patients with acute pulmonary embolism and right ventricular dysfunction, but without hypotension ("submassive PE"), should be considered for thrombolysis on a case-by-case basis, informed by clinical risk of hemodynamic decompensation as well as risk factors for bleeding.
- Accelerated regimens of thrombolytic therapy, concomitant with expert management of heparin anticoagulation, reduce thrombotic burden, decrease pulmonary artery pressures, and improve mortality in the right clinical setting.

INTRODUCTION

The risks of hemodynamically significant pulmonary embolism (PE) are substantial. The estimated 30-day case-fatality rate from PE ranges from 10% to 30%,[1–4] with most PE-related deaths occurring within the first day of presentation.[5] PE presenting

[a] Department of Medicine, University Health Network and Sinai Health System, University of Toronto, 585 University Avenue, 7th Floor, Room 739, Toronto, Ontario M5G 2N2, Canada; [b] Ottawa Blood Disease Centre, The Ottawa Hospital, Ottawa, Canada; [c] Department of Medicine, St. Joseph's Healthcare Hamilton, McMaster University, 50 Charlton Avenue East, F: 403, Hamilton, Ontario L8N 4A6, Canada
* Corresponding author.
E-mail address: eric.kaplovitch@uhn.ca
Twitter: @kaplovitch (E.K.)

Crit Care Clin 36 (2020) 465–480
https://doi.org/10.1016/j.ccc.2020.02.004
0749-0704/20/© 2020 Elsevier Inc. All rights reserved.

criticalcare.theclinics.com

with shock carries an approximate 25% risk of mortality, whereas PE requiring cardiopulmonary resuscitation carries a tremendous 65% mortality.[6]

In clinical practice today, morbidity and mortality from PE arise from the cardiopulmonary implications of PE as well as the side effects, namely bleeding, of aggressive treatment. Even if the patient survives the acute hazards of a large PE, chronic thromboembolic pulmonary hypertension can manifest as a debilitating sequela.[7] The use of thrombolytic agents has therefore been widely investigated, despite their bleeding risks, in order to curb the malignant nature of high-risk thromboembolic disease.

Multiple metaanalyses have aggregated clinical trial data over the last 5 decades for thrombolysis in PE, but have come to disparate conclusions.[8–10] The discrepancy likely comes from heterogeneity between small trials using different doses and formulations of thrombolytic agents as well as investigating patients with different baseline risk of decompensation and death.

Understanding the evidence base, the nuanced stratification of a patient's hemodynamic and bleeding risk, as well the practical considerations for administering thrombolysis, allows the critical care practitioner to choose appropriate candidates for thrombolysis and optimally administer this therapy.

RATIONALE FOR THROMBOLYSIS

The potential for thrombolysis was discovered in 1933, when a substance isolated from group A streptococcus, originally termed streptococcal fibrinolysin and later shortened to streptokinase, was found to rapidly liquefy clotted fibrin of normal human plasma.[11,12] Thirty-five years later, the first report of systemic thrombolysis was successfully used for acute myocardial infarction.[13] Extrapolating to the similar thrombotic pathophysiology of acute PE, Sautter and colleagues[14] described the first successful cohort of PE patients treated with thrombolysis in 1967, demonstrating excellent clinical response with noted radiographic and hemodynamic response to therapy (**Fig. 1**). In the wake of this and similar[15–17] observations, uptake of thrombolysis for PE increased, with varying formulations receiving approval from governing bodies guiding medication use.[18,19]

The pathophysiologic basis for thrombolysis is robust and concordant with clinical, hemodynamic, and radiologic observations. Acute PE causes an abrupt increase in pulmonary vascular resistance and right ventricular (RV) afterload, mediated by physical obstruction of the pulmonary arteries as well as hypoxemia and release of pulmonary artery (PA) vasoconstrictors.[20] This increase in RV afterload translates to RV dilation as well as increased RV myocardial demand, resulting in RV infarction, ultimately leading to frank RV failure.[21] Simultaneously, given ventricular interdependence, dilation of the right ventricle bows the interventricular septum to the left, decreasing left ventricular preload.[21] In the case of massive PE, a cycle of RV damage and RV dysfunction self-perpetuates, leading to shock and ultimately cardiac arrest (**Fig. 2**).[20,21] Hypoxia is a result of the combination of ventilation to perfusion mismatch, increase in dead space, and at times right-to-left shunt (either because of atelectasis or across the foramen ovale as right atrial pressure exceeds left atrial pressure).[20,22] The balance of hypoxia and hemodynamic instability is ultimately dependent on the size and distribution of PE as well as the patient's underlying cardiorespiratory reserve.

Thrombolytic agents bind to fibrin within a thrombus and convert the entrapped plasminogen to plasmin, thereby initiating fibrinolysis locally with limited systemic proteolysis. Thrombolysis aids in the rapid dissolution of pulmonary thrombus,[23,24] with an associated rapid decrease in PA pressures as compared with those treated with

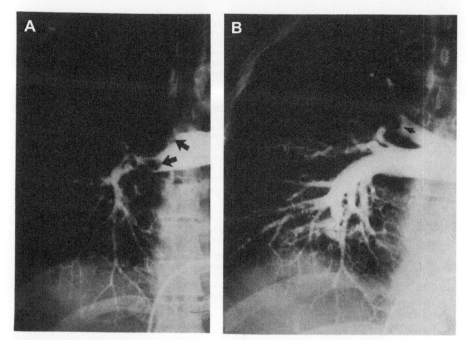

Fig. 1. Pulmonary arteriogram before and after recombinant tissue-type plasminogen activator (rt-PA) treatment in a patient with massive PE. Initial pulmonary arteriogram (*A*) showing large embolus in the main right pulmonary artery causing complete occlusion of the right upper lobe branch and partial occlusion of the right middle and right lower lobe branches (*arrows*), with (*B*) marked resolution following rt-PA treatment. (*From* Goldhaber SZ, Meyerovitz MF, Markis JE, et al. Thrombolytic therapy of acute pulmonary embolism: current status and future potential. J Am Coll Cardiol 1987;10(5 supplement 2):96B-104B; with permission.)

heparin alone.[23] This decrease in PA pressure interrupts the downward spiral toward cardiac decompensation, with thrombolysis shown to rapidly decrease RV diameter, improve RV function, increase LV diameter, and result in more favorable hemodynamics.[24]

THE EVOLVING EVIDENCE FOR THROMBOLYSIS

Risk of morbidity or mortality is heterogeneous within PE presentations. Only those at the highest thrombotic risk, namely those with "massive" or "submassive" PE, merit consideration of a hazardous intervention such as thrombolysis. Originally based on angiographic rather than clinical findings,[25] the definitions of both massive and submassive PE have been varied and ambiguous.[26] Practically, and most commonly, massive PE refers to those with acute PE and either persistent systemic arterial hypotension or cardiac arrest.[18,19,26–28] Similarly, submassive PE has had varying definitions, but generally refers to acute PE with evidence of RV injury or dysfunction, but without systemic arterial hypotension.[18,19,27,28] Although thrombolytics are approved by the Food and Drug Administration (FDA) for the treatment of massive PE,[19] increasing evidence and experience have led to more liberal use of thrombolysis for patients with submassive PE.[29]

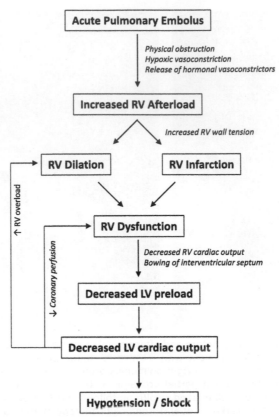

Fig. 2. Pathophysiology of massive PE. LV, left ventricular. (*Adapted from* Lualdi JC, Goldhaber SZ. Right ventricular dysfunction after acute pulmonary embolism: Pathophysiologic factors, detection, and therapeutic implications. *Am Heart J*. 1995;130(6):1276-1282.)

MASSIVE PULMONARY EMBOLISM

Given the life-threatening nature of massive PE, and that immediate intervention is often required, conducting large randomized controlled trials on the highest-risk PE syndromes can be difficult. Moreover, published trials include heterogenous patient populations with discrepant PE risk profiles, use varying thrombolytic agents and doses, and have varying outcome definitions.

The first randomized controlled trial for thrombolysis in PE, the Urokinase Pulmonary Embolism Trial (UPET), randomized patients with acute PE to a bolus and 12-hour infusion of urokinase, with subsequent heparin, versus heparin alone.[24] Study inclusion was highly heterogeneous, including patients with as little PE burden as 1 segmental PA.[24] Only 9% of patients exhibited hemodynamically significant (massive) PE.[24] It was therefore unsurprising that although urokinase significantly accelerated the resolution rate of pulmonary thromboemboli at 24 hours as shown by pulmonary arteriograms, lung radiography, and right-sided pressure measurements, it failed to demonstrate mortality benefit within the 2 weeks of follow-up (urokinase: 7.3% vs heparin: 8.9%).[24] The investigators noted however that those with poor cardiac index or pulmonary arteriography score at baseline gained the most improvement from systemic thrombolysis, the latter demonstrating a 33.4% to 68.6% radiographic improvement, compared with a 6.2% improvement with heparin alone.[24] Bleeding complications manifested in 45% of patients receiving urokinase and 27% receiving heparin alone, largely occurring within the first 24 hours of therapy, with the difference almost exclusively manifesting at sites of intervention (venous cut-down, and so forth).[24] The inference was that thrombolysis may be of benefit in patients at highest risk of decompensation and death, whereby the risk of moderate to severe bleeding is outweighed by hemodynamic improvement.

In the wake of UPET, other small, heterogenous studies similarly demonstrated angiographic improvement or hemodynamic improvement but were underpowered to detect a difference in mortality.[30,31] Ly and colleagues[31] demonstrated significant angiographic improvement ($P<.01$) with a bolus and 72-hour infusion streptokinase regimen compared with heparin alone, although at the expense of numerically increased bleeding (28.6% vs 18.2%). The investigation of Dotter and colleagues[30] of bolus and maintenance (18–72 hours) streptokinase in combination with heparin, versus heparin alone, analogously showed significantly improved angiographic extent of PE ($P<.0125$), with no significant increase in bleeding (streptokinase 20% vs heparin 25%). Importantly, 6 of 7 major bleeding events within the streptokinase group were related to invasive procedures rather than spontaneous events.[30]

Through the 1980s, the predominant consensus was that systemic thrombolysis clearly improved the hemodynamics and thrombotic burden in PE patients, but at the cost of increased bleeding. Mortality benefit was therefore inferred to those at highest risk of death. In light of this continued equipoise, a 40-patient randomized controlled trial was planned, investigating a 1-hour, 1,500,000-IU regimen of strepto-kinase followed by heparin, versus heparin alone, in the treatment of massive PE.[32] The first 8 patients all presented in cardiogenic shock.[32] All 4 patients randomized to heparin alone died within 3 hours of hospitalization.[32] All 4 patients randomized to streptokinase survived to 2-year follow-up (mortality 100% vs 0%; $P = .02$).[32] The streptokinase group had rapid improvement in symptoms, heart rate, diastolic blood pressure, oxygenation, as well as a large immediate drop in PA systolic pressure (prestreptokinase: 97 ± 4.76; 1-hour after streptokinase: 32 ± 4.08).[32] Remarkably, all 4 streptokinase patients were without pulmonary hypertension at 2-year follow-up.[32] The main confounder in this trial was the earlier presentation to hospital following symptom onset for the streptokinase group (2.50 ± 1.29 hour) as opposed to the hep-arin group (34.75 ± 19.35 hour). There was however similar time from onset of cardio-genic shock to time of intervention (streptokinase: 2.25 ± 0.50 hour; heparin: 1.75 ± 0.96 hour).[32] In light of these preliminary results, the trial was terminated early, and the use of systemic thrombolysis has since been a key component in the manage-ment of high-risk pulmonary emboli.

Metaanalyses of the trials including massive PE are challenging, because the overall number of patients included are small, and most contributing studies do not report outcomes specific to unstable patients. An early metaanalysis demonstrated that thrombolytic therapy for hemodynamically significant PE significantly decreased the composite of recurrent PE or death (9.4% vs 19.0%; odds ratio [OR]: 0.45; 95% con-fidence interval [CI]: 0.22–0.92).[33] A later metaanalysis, investigating the outcome of death alone, showed a strong but insignificant trend to improved survival (OR: 0.48; CI: 0.20–1.15).[9] The heterogeneous inclusion of nonmassive PE likely underestimates the effect of thrombolysis on survival in true hemodynamically unstable PE. Real-world experience with massive PE, investigated using the Nationwide Inpatient Sample Cohort in the United States, demonstrated that the case fatality attributable to massive PE was 8.4% in those treated with thrombolytic as opposed to 42% in those treated with anticoagulant alone (relative risk [RR]: 0.20; 95% CI: 0.19–0.22; $P<.0001$).[34]

Despite widespread acceptance of thrombolysis for massive PE at the time of study, only 30% of hemodynamically unstable patients received such therapy.[34]

Guidelines are consistent that thrombolytics should be used in clinically massive PE. Patients with acute PE and hypotension (systolic blood pressure <90 mm Hg for 15 minutes), vasopressor requirements, cardiac arrest, or malignant bradycardia should receive systemically administered thrombolytics.[18,19,27,35] Early intervention with thrombolytic therapy has therefore become the standard of care. Despite this, it is prudent to recognize that each society appropriately states a caveat based on bleeding risk. Those with contraindications (**Fig. 3**) may be best served by alternative therapy to systemic thrombolysis. The decision to proceed with thrombolysis and selection of the route of administration must be individualized based on hemodynamic and bleeding considerations.[18,19,27,35]

SUBMASSIVE PULMONARY EMBOLISM

The use of thrombolysis in submassive PE continues to evolve. Although most of the earlier trials in PE included submassive phenotypes of disease, the earliest study dedicated to hemodynamically stable patients with RV dysfunction was published by Goldhaber and colleagues[36] in 1993. In those with baseline RV dysfunction following acute PE, a 100-mg infusion of alteplase followed by heparin was more effective than heparin alone in improving RV hemodynamics (89% improved vs 44% improved; $P = .03$). Most patients experienced benefit within 3 hours of infusion.[36] A numerically greater number of patients randomized to alteplase survived 2 weeks of follow-up (18/18 vs 16/18).[36] These results, coupled with pathophysiologic plausibility, triggered a call for investigations in submassive PE with a focus on clinical outcomes.

American College of Chest Physicians	American Heart Association	European Society of Cardiology
Major Contraindications	**Absolute Contraindications**	**Absolute Contraindications**
Previous intracranial hemorrhage	Previous intracranial hemorrhage	Previous hemorrhagic stroke or stroke of unknown origin
Structural intracranial disease	Structural intracranial disease	Central nervous system damage or neoplasms
Ischemic stroke within 3 mo	Ischemic stroke within 3 mo	Ischemic stroke within 6 mo
Active bleeding	Suspected aortic dissection	GI bleeding within 1 mo
Bleeding diathesis	Active bleeding or bleeding diathesis	Recent major trauma, surgery, or head injury in the preceding 3 wk
Recent brain or spinal surgery	Recent surgery encroaching on the spinal canal or brain	Known bleeding risk
Recent head trauma with fracture or brain injury	Recent closed-head or facial trauma with radiographic evidence of bony fracture or brain injury	
Relative Contraindications	**Relative Contraindications**	**Relative Contraindications**
Age >75 y	Age >75 y	TIA in preceding 6 mo
Anticoagulant therapy	Anticoagulant therapy	Anticoagulant therapy
Pregnancy	Pregnancy	Pregnancy
Recent invasive procedure	Noncompressible vascular punctures	Noncompressible puncture site
Traumatic CPR	Traumatic or prolonged CPR (>10 min)	Traumatic resuscitation
Recent non-intracranial bleeding	Recent internal bleeding (within 2 to 4 wk)	Active peptic ulcer disease
Pericarditis or pericardial fluid	Chronic, poorly controlled HTN	Infective endocarditis
Systolic BP >180 or Diastolic BP >110	Systolic BP >180 or diastolic BP >110	Refractory hypertension (systolic BP >180)
Weight <60 kg	Dementia	Advanced liver disease
Ischemic stroke > 3 mo ago	Ischemic stroke > 3 mo ago	
Recent surgery	Major surgery within 3 wk	
Diabetic retinopathy		
Female		
Black race		

Fig. 3. Contraindications to thrombolysis according to societal guideline. CPR, cardiopulmonary resuscitation; GI, gastrointestinal: HTN, hypertension; TIA, transient ischemic attack.

The MAPPET-3 trial investigated patients with acute PE without systemic hypotension, but with either RV dysfunction or pulmonary hypertension. Patients were randomized to alteplase 10-mg bolus and 90-mg infusion over 2 hours versus placebo, with concomitant heparin infusion targeting usual anticoagulation.[37] Those randomized to heparin with placebo were significantly more likely to reach the primary endpoint of in-hospital death or clinical deterioration requiring escalation of treatment (placebo: 24.6% vs 11.0%; P = .006), although overall mortality remained similar between the 2 groups (2.2% vs 3.4%; P = .71).[37] The difference in primary endpoint was largely accounted for by the increased need for rescue thrombolysis in the placebo group (23.2% vs 7.6%; P = .001).[37] Unexpectedly, however, bleeding risk was quite low in both groups (3.6% vs 0.8%; P = .29),[37] perhaps attributable to lower rates of invasive procedures as compared with previous trials. The trial was stopped early because of its positive interim analysis, potentially exaggerating findings on the 1 hand, but also resulted in insufficient power to detect a more clinically meaningful difference in mortality.

Until this point, conclusions regarding mortality benefit and thrombolysis for submassive PE were unclear at best. Fasullo and colleagues[38] mirrored the MAPPET-3 trial, using bolus (10 mg) and infusion (90 mg over 2 hours) alteplase versus placebo in patients receiving heparin for submassive PE, but included only those with confirmed echocardiographic RV dysfunction. The result was a more hemodynamically unstable patient population, clinically apparent as well, given lower baseline blood pressure and higher heart rate at inclusion.[37,38] Although thrombolysis demonstrated significantly faster improvement in all echocardiographic hemodynamics at 24 hours, the trial is most noted for its clinical outcomes.[38] Patients randomized to alteplase experienced significantly decreased in-hospital death (0% vs 17.1%; P = .027).[38] Adverse thrombotic or bleeding events were infrequent after discharge.[38]

The Tenecteplase Or Placebo: Cardiopulmonary Outcomes At Three months (TOPCOAT) trial investigated single-tiered bolus of tenecteplase or placebo, in addition to low-molecular-weight heparin (LMWH), in hemodynamically stable patients with RV strain.[39] Although baseline echocardiography was included in study protocol, qualification for study could be achieved by either hypokinesis on echocardiography, elevated troponin above the 99th percentile, or elevation in brain natriuretic protein (BNP >90 pg/nL or pro-BNP >900 pg/nL).[39] Most patients were included based on biochemical evidence of RV dysfunction/injury rather than echocardiographic findings.[39] Similar in-hospital mortality was noted between the thrombolysis and placebo groups.[39] The study arms truly diverged with respect to functional outcomes at 90-day follow-up.[39] Patients treated with placebo had a numerically higher chance of poor functional capacity at 90 days (8/43 vs 4/40), low perception of wellness (9/43 vs 1/40), and recurrent VTE (4/43 vs 1/40).[39] Including both early and late adverse outcomes, patients treated with tenecteplase were 22% more likely to have event-free survival at 90 days (22%; CI: 3.2%–40%; P = .017).[39] Previous investigations had largely focused on immediate outcomes following thrombolysis, a reasonable strategy given the high immediate morbidity and mortality following massive or submassive PE. Although physiologically intuitive, TOPCOAT demonstrated the downstream effects of thrombolysis, raising the possibility that acute decisions regarding clot dissolution have longstanding implications for cardiopulmonary function and quality of life. In the process, TOPCOAT further expanded the definition of submassive PE, using increasingly available cardiac biomarkers, troponin and BNP, to aid in risk stratification.

The Pulmonary Embolism Thrombolysis (PEITHO) trial represents the largest trial to date investigating thrombolysis in submassive PE, randomizing patients to a weight-based bolus of tenecteplase (30–50 mg) versus placebo in addition to standard heparin.[40] In an effort to identify patients with a high degree of aberrant cardiac physiology, PEITHO required both RV dysfunction on echocardiography and myocardial injury (elevated troponin) for inclusion. However, the mean clinical characteristics of the PEITHO study population were not consistent with a particularly unstable cohort, given a mean systolic blood pressure greater than 130 mm Hg and a mean baseline heart rate of less than 95 beats per minute. Although thrombolysis decreased the primary composite outcome of death and hemodynamic decompensation at 7 days (OR: 0.44; CI: 0.23–0.87; P = .22), this result was largely driven by decreased decompensation (OR: 0.30; CI: 0.14–0.68; P = .002) rather than an impact on mortality.[40] The improvement in hemodynamics came at the expense of significantly increased major extracranial bleeding (OR: 5.55; CI: 2.3–13.39; $P<.001$) as well as hemorrhagic or ischemic stroke (OR: 12.10; CI: 1.57–93.39; P = .003).[40] Overall, tenecteplase treatment resulted in numerically lower (1.2% vs 1.8%), but statistically insignificant, differences in overall mortality (OR: 0.65; CI: 0.23–1.85; P = .42).[40] A noteworthy trend was improved efficacy and lower bleeding risk in patients aged less than 75, although these findings did not achieve statistical significance.[40]

Catheter-Based Thrombolysis for Submassive Pulmonary Embolism

Because hemodynamic benefits of thrombolysis are counterbalanced by bleeding complications, there has been increasing investigation into catheter-directed thrombolysis, with the thought of minimizing the dose of thrombolytic and administering a high concentration of therapy proximate to thrombus. Studies to date however have been small and largely observational.

The Ultrasound Accelerated Thrombolysis of Pulmonary Embolism (ULTIMA) trial is the most robust randomized controlled trial of catheter-based intervention in submassive PE.[41] Randomizing 59 hemodynamically stable patients with RV dilation to a 15-hour infusion of catheter-guided alteplase (10–20 mg) in addition to heparin, versus heparin alone, ULTIMA demonstrated significant improvement in cardiac dynamics ($P<.001$).[41] Because patients were hemodynamically low risk (mean HR = 87, mean systolic blood pressure = 134), adverse clinical outcomes were uncommon.[41] At 90 days, there were no cases of hemodynamic decompensation or major bleeding events.[41] One death occurred overall, in a patient randomized to heparin, but as a consequence of pancreatic cancer rather than thrombotic or bleeding complications.[41]

Drawing definitive conclusions from the numerous small observational studies evaluating catheter-directed thrombolysis is difficult because of heterogeneity with respect to techniques used, patient populations, and study quality.[42] Narrative reviews summarizing the findings from these small studies seem to suggest that the bleeding rate for catheter-directed thrombolysis is lower than systemic therapy, although direct comparisons cannot be made because of differences in the underlying populations.[43] Conversely, these techniques are associated with complications directly attributable to the invasive nature of the intervention, such as pulmonary hemorrhage, perforation or dissection of a major PA, pericardial tamponade, and arrythmias.

Approach to the Management of Submassive Pulmonary Embolism

Thrombolysis in submassive PE reverses aberrant cardiac physiology and therefore improves hemodynamics, but comes at an expectedly higher bleeding rate. Metaanalyses comparing thrombolysis to anticoagulation in submassive PE differ with respect to their conclusions surrounding mortality, depending on the trials included and the statistical techniques used.[8–10] Only the most liberally inclusive metaanalysis of thrombolysis in submassive PE demonstrated a significant decrease in overall mortality (OR: 0.48; CI: 0.25–0.92), with small absolute differences (1.39% vs 2.92%), and an increase in major bleeding (OR: 3.19; 95% CI: 2.07–4.92).[10] In this metaanalysis, statistical significance was maintained with respect to mortality and bleeding outcomes following a sensitivity analysis that excluded investigations for catheter-based therapies.[10]

In clinical practice, the net benefit of thrombolysis for PE likely exists on a continuum, highly dependent on the severity of the clinical presentation, a patient's comorbidities, and bleeding risk, as well as availability of alternative therapies. Varying guidelines and consensus statements convey differing approaches to risk stratification, largely based on echocardiographic features and cardiac biomarkers (troponin and BNP).[18,19,27,35] Interestingly, cardiac biomarkers prove to be particularly predictive of PE-related death,[44] with mortality in hemodynamically stable PE best prognosticated by BNP (OR: 9.51; CI: 3.16–28.64), troponin elevation (OR: 8.31; CI: 3.57–21.49), echocardiography (OR: 2.53; CI: 1.17–5.50), and computed tomography (OR: 2.29; CI: 0.87–5.98) in descending order.[45]

Although the evolving evidence for submassive PE has shifted the use of thrombolysis to less acute presentations, the routine use of thrombolysis in this setting should be avoided.[27] Caution is strongly advised in patients with radiologically large, but clinically low-risk PE. Because original classifications for PE were based on anatomic distribution of thrombus,[25] radiology reports may describe "massive" PE in patients without hemodynamic concerns and minimal hypoxia. There are similar reports of incidental, "radiologically massive," or saddle PEs in asymptomatic patients.[46] An individualized approach to thrombolysis is essential, not only based on radiologic or biochemical findings but also with a heavy emphasis on the patient's clinical status. It is unsurprising that the trial of Fasullo and colleagues[38] included arguably the most hemodynamically unwell patients and resulted as the only individual trial to demonstrate mortality benefit. Patients with submassive PE deemed to be at high risk of decompensation and death, considered based on the totality of the clinical picture, should be considered for thrombolysis, particularly if deemed to be at low risk of bleeding complications. Given the state of the evidence for catheter-directed thrombolysis, clinical guidelines recognize that catheterization cannot be recommended routinely over systemic administration of lytic therapy.[18,27,35] Catheter-based strategies remain useful tools in equipped centers for patients with concomitant high hemodynamic risk and high bleeding risk. Patient counseling on absolute risks and benefits (**Table 1**) before proceeding with any form of thrombolysis is essential.

PRACTICAL CONSIDERATIONS IN THROMBOLYSIS

Practical aspects surrounding the administration of thrombolytic agents can be challenging. The timing of therapy, choice of agent and dosing, identification of contraindications, and management of anticoagulation can lead to difficult decisions even for an experienced critical care physician.

Three different thrombolytics have FDA approval for the treatment of PE (**Table 2**): urokinase as a 4400-IU/kg intravenous (IV) bolus, followed by a 4400-IU/kg/h infusion over 12 to 24 hours; streptokinase via a 250,000-IU IV loading dose over 30 minutes, followed by 100,000 IU/h over 12 to 24 hours, and alteplase as a 100-mg IV infusion over 2 hours, without bolus.[18,19,47] Despite the historical use of prolonged infusions, contemporary evidence demonstrates that accelerated thrombolysis may have more favorable outcomes. Shorter regimens, namely 2 hours or less, are associated

Table 1
Risks and benefits of systemic thrombolysis versus anticoagulation for acute PE[a]

	Thrombolysis (%)	Anticoagulation Alone (%)	Relative Effect	Number Needed to Treat or Harm
All-cause mortality	2.17	3.89	OR: 0.53 (0.32–0.88)	NNT = 59
Major bleeding	9.24	3.42	OR: 2.73 (1.91–3.91)	NNH = 18
Intracranial hemorrhage	1.46	0.19	OR: 4.63 (1.78–12.04)	NNH = 78
Recurrent PE	1.17	3.04	OR: 0.40 (0.22–0.74)	NNT = 54

Abbreviations: NNH, number needed to harm; NNT, number needed to treat.
[a] Vast majority (83%) of patient population included suffered submassive PE. Low-risk PE included in estimate as well. Absolute risks are definitively higher in massive PE. Contemporary observational data have suggested a case fatality rate of 8.4% in those treated with thrombolysis as opposed to 42% treated without thrombolysis (RR 0.20; 95% CI, 0.19–0.22; $P<.0001$).[34]
Adapted from Chatterjee S, Chakraborty A, Weinberg I, et al. Thrombolysis for pulmonary embolism and risk of all-cause mortality, major bleeding, and intracranial hemorrhage: A meta-analysis. *JAMA.* 2014;311(23):2414-2421 and Kearon C, Akl EA, Ornelas J, et al. Antithrombotic therapy for VTE disease: CHEST guideline and expert panel report. *Chest.* 2016;149(2):315-352.

with lower bleeding rates, more rapid clot lysis, and at least equivalent clinical outcomes when compared with infusion regimens of 12 hours or longer.[28] Accelerated regimens of thrombolytic are therefore often used in clinical practice. Urokinase is often administered as a 3-million IU infusion over 2 hours, whereas streptokinase is often administered as a 1.5-million IU infusion over 2 hours.[18]

Alteplase is the most commonly administered thrombolytic. Although the FDA-approved dose of 100 mg of alteplase over 2 hours is most commonly used, there is evidence that this regimen may be improved on as well. Based on animal models demonstrating that short infusions of alteplase achieve sufficient local thrombolysis while minimizing systemic lytic activity, it was postulated that a short bolus of reduced-dose alteplase would be more effective at resolving PEs while causing less bleeding.[48] After demonstrating physiologic efficacy versus placebo,[48] reduced bolus alteplase at a dose of 0.6 mg/kg (to a maximum of 50 mg) has been compared with the usual 2-hour alteplase infusion.[49–51] Metaanalyses of this strategy demonstrated similar efficacy between the 2 regimens.[52,53] Moreover, there is at least a strong trend toward lower rates of bleeding with reduced-dose alteplase, with 1 metaanalysis demonstrating a significant benefit.[52] Reduced-dose alteplase has also been shown to be associated with lower laboratory markers of systematic fibrinolytic activation.[49] There seems to be particular benefit for low-dose alteplase in those with low body weight.[51] Although not explicitly addressed in the latest American thrombosis guideline,[27] European and Canadian guidance supports the option of alteplase 0.6 mg/kg (up to 50 mg) administered over 15 minutes.[18,35] In the case of impending or actual cardiac arrest, any agent of thrombolysis should be given as a bolus when possible.[28]

The decision regarding thrombolysis is not only dependent on the efficacy of therapy but also tied to a patient's estimated bleeding risk. Absolute and relative contraindications are published throughout various guidelines (see **Fig. 3**). Given the heterogeneity of clinical trials, however, these contraindications are largely extrapolated from the literature surrounding myocardial infarction.[19] Absolute contraindications should preclude systemic thrombolysis, and save for extenuating circumstances, should prompt strong consideration for alternative methods of

Table 2
Thrombolytic regimens for acute pulmonary embolus

Alteplase[a]		Streptokinase[a]		Urokinase[a]		Reteplase	Tenecteplase
Classical Regimen	Accelerated Regimen	Classical Regimen	Accelerated Regimen	Classical Regimen	Accelerated Regimen		
100 mg infusion over 2 h	0.6 mg/kg (up to 50 mg) bolus over 15 min	250,000 IU bolus over 30 min, followed by 100,000 IU/h over 12–24 h	1.5 million IU infusion over 2 h	4400 IU/kg bolus, followed by 4400 IU/ kg/h infusion over 12–24 h	3 million IU infusion over 2 h	Two boluses of 10 units given 30 min apart	Weight-based bolus over 5 s: <60 kg: 30 mg ≥60 to <70 kg: 35 mg ≥70 to <80 kg: 40 mg ≥80 to <90 kg: 45 mg ≥90 kg: 50 mg

[a] FDA approved thrombolytic for PE.

thrombus removal. Relative contraindications should be interpreted as precautions rather stand-alone reasons to avoid thrombolytic treatment. Clearly, female sex, age ≥75, and black race, identified as relative contraindications by the most recent American College of Chest Physicians guidelines, should not exclude therapy in the right clinical circumstance.[27] These contraindications can be best thought of as risk factors, increasing the RR of bleeding and perhaps changing the calculus in offering thrombolysis when there is equipoise as to utility. Observational studies show that patients with ≥5 of these precautions have an intracranial bleeding risk of 4.1%, as opposed to an intracranial bleed risk of 0.7% in those with ≤1 risk factors.[27] It therefore stands to reason that the risk of bleeding even in those with multiple precautions is likely outweighed by ischemic risk in massive PE, which is accompanied by upwards of 25% mortality risk.[6] Although age as a risk factor is dichotomized at 75 years, it is best thought of as a continuous variable, with an approximately 4% increase in major bleeding risk for each additional year of age.[27,54] Modifiable risk factors for bleeding, such as elevated blood pressure, should be treated where possible. Overall, although risk factors for bleeding are essential to consider, individualized clinical judgment must be used to most effectively weigh risks and benefits.

This decision for thrombolysis is best reached on an expedited basis. Although benefit of thrombolysis extends until at least 14 days from symptom onset, efficacy significantly diminishes with each passing day.[55] A movement to create pulmonary embolism response teams (PERTs) is growing within North America in order to facilitate complex decision making from multiple involved specialists. Similar to the ubiquitous ST-elevation myocardial infarction teams or stroke teams, PERTs function to deliver rapid multidisciplinary, life-saving interventions.[56]

Once a decision for thrombolysis has been made, careful management of parenteral anticoagulation is prudent. Because of the high risk of bleeding associated with thrombolysis, and the potential need for immediate reversal in the case of life-threatening hemorrhage, unfractionated heparin (UFH) is often the preferred anticoagulant to be given concomitantly to thrombolysis. Exceptionally high doses of heparin are often required in massive PE. The management of UFH infusion during thrombolysis varies by location. In the United States, UFH is often held during thrombolytic infusion, whereas European guidelines advocate for continued UFH during alteplase specifically.[18] Practice is variable by site and practitioner. If the decision is made to hold anticoagulation, UFH should be restarted at the same infusion rate as before thrombolysis, without bolus, once the activated partial thromboplastin time is ≤80 seconds (or less than twice the normal value).[28,47] Practically, this can be challenging. Moreover, maintaining therapeutic anticoagulation is essential in the high-risk period following thrombolysis, because physiologically, a rebound accumulation of fibrin on thrombi is apparent immediately after thrombolytic infusion.[57] Continuing UFH during bolus thrombolysis regimens in particular seems prudent to avoid logistical errors and subtherapeutic anticoagulation.

Although UFH is the preferred anticoagulant around the time of thrombolysis, there is clinical experience, and clinical trial experience,[39] in performing thrombolysis following LMWH. If thrombolysis is administered in this setting, LMWH should be switched to UFH at the next scheduled LMWH dose (ie, 12 hours after a twice daily dose or 24 hours following a once daily dose). There is a paucity of experience with thrombolysis while on direct oral anticoagulants (DOACs). Logically, recent administration of a DOAC should not prevent thrombolytic therapy in emergent situations such as impending or actual cardiac arrest. However, these patients should likely be transitioned to UFH at the time of the next scheduled dose of DOAC, for the reasons mentions above.

SUMMARY

Thrombolysis is an increasingly important tool in a critical care physician's armamentarium. PE with hemodynamic instability or RV impairment is not uncommon and remains associated with high morbidity and mortality. Thrombolysis has become the standard of care in patients with massive PE, unless excessive bleeding risk prohibits therapy. Submassive PE represents a heterogenous clinical entity, making consideration for thrombolysis dependent on individualized hemodynamic and bleeding risk. Although radiologic, biochemical, and echocardiographic features can aid practitioners in the decision for thrombolysis, consideration of clinical status is paramount. Further studies will be invaluable in clarifying the role of catheter-instilled thrombolysis for PE. Ultimately, a conscientious approach to thrombolysis and expert management of thrombolytic agents allow the critical care physician to prevent hemodynamic decompensation and death in patients at highest risk of clinical deterioration.

REFERENCES

1. Kroger K, Moerchel C, Moysidis T, et al. Incidence rate of pulmonary embolism in Germany: data from the Federal Statistical Office. J Thromb Thrombolysis 2010; 29(3):349–53.
2. Wiener RS, Schwartz LM, Woloshin S. Time trends in pulmonary embolism in the United States: evidence of overdiagnosis. Arch Intern Med 2011;171(9):831–7.
3. Beckman MG, Hooper WC, Critchley SE, et al. Venous thromboembolism: a public health concern. Am J Prev Med 2010;38(4 Suppl):S495–501.
4. Cushman M, Tsai AW, White RH, et al. Deep vein thrombosis and pulmonary embolism in two cohorts: the longitudinal investigation of thromboembolism etiology. Am J Med 2004;117(1):19–25.
5. Heit JA, Silverstein MD, Mohr DN, et al. Predictors of survival after deep vein thrombosis and pulmonary embolism: a population-based, cohort study. Arch Intern Med 1999;159(5):445–53.
6. Kasper W, Konstantinides S, Geibel A, et al. Management strategies and determinants of outcome in acute major pulmonary embolism: results of a multicenter registry. J Am Coll Cardiol 1997;30(5):1165–71.
7. Fanikos J, Piazza G, Zayaruzny M, et al. Long-term complications of medical patients with hospital-acquired venous thromboembolism. Thromb Haemost 2009; 102(4):688–93.
8. Nakamura S, Takano H, Kubota Y, et al. Impact of the efficacy of thrombolytic therapy on the mortality of patients with acute submassive pulmonary embolism: a meta-analysis. J Thromb Haemost 2014;12(7):1086–95.
9. Marti C, John G, Konstantinides S, et al. Systemic thrombolytic therapy for acute pulmonary embolism: a systematic review and meta-analysis. Eur Heart J 2015; 36(10):605–14.
10. Chatterjee S, Chakraborty A, Weinberg I, et al. Thrombolysis for pulmonary embolism and risk of all-cause mortality, major bleeding, and intracranial hemorrhage: a meta-analysis. JAMA 2014;311(23):2414–21.
11. Sherry S. The origin of thrombolytic therapy. J Am Coll Cardiol 1989;14(4): 1085–92.
12. Tillett WS, Garner RL. The fibrinolytic activity of hemolytic streptococci. J Exp Med 1933;58(4):485–502.
13. Fletcher AP, Alkjaersig N, Smyrniotis FE, et al. The treatment of patients suffering from early myocardial infarction with massive and prolonged streptokinase therapy. Trans Assoc Am Physicians 1958;71:287–96.

14. Sautter RD, Emanuel DA, Fletcher FW, et al. Urokinase for the treatment of acute pulmonary thromboembolism. JAMA 1967;202(3):215–8.
15. Tow DE, Wagner HN, Holmes RA. Urokinase in pulnonary embolism. N Engl J Med 1967;277(22):1161–7.
16. Sasahara AA, Cannilla JE, Belko JS, et al. Urokinase therapy in clinical pulmonary embolism. A new thrombolytic agent. N Engl J Med 1967;277(22):1168–73.
17. Genton E, Wolf PS. Urokinase therapy in pulmonary thromboembolism. Am Heart J 1968;76(5):628–37.
18. Konstantinides SV, Torbicki A, Agnelli G, et al. 2014 ESC guidelines on the diagnosis and management of acute pulmonary embolism. Eur Heart J 2014;35(43): 3033–69, 3069a-3069k.
19. Jaff MR, McMurtry MS, Archer SL, et al. Management of massive and submassive pulmonary embolism, iliofemoral deep vein thrombosis, and chronic thromboembolic pulmonary hypertension: a scientific statement from the American Heart Association. Circulation 2011;123(16):1788–830.
20. Goldhaber SZ, Elliott CG. Acute pulmonary embolism: part I: epidemiology, pathophysiology, and diagnosis. Circulation 2003;108(22):2726–9.
21. Lualdi JC, Goldhaber SZ. Right ventricular dysfunction after acute pulmonary embolism: pathophysiologic factors, detection, and therapeutic implications. Am Heart J 1995;130(6):1276–82.
22. Elliott CG. Pulmonary physiology during pulmonary embolism. Chest 1992;101(4 Suppl):163S–71S.
23. Dalla-Volta S, Palla A, Santolicandro A, et al. PAIMS 2: alteplase combined with heparin versus heparin in the treatment of acute pulmonary embolism. Plasminogen Activator Italian Multicenter Study 2. J Am Coll Cardiol 1992;20(3):520–6.
24. Urokinase pulmonary embolism trial. Phase 1 results: a cooperative study. JAMA 1970;214(12):2163–72.
25. Miller GA, Sutton GC, Kerr IH, et al. Comparison of streptokinase and heparin in treatment of isolated acute massive pulmonary embolism. Br Med J 1971; 2(5763):681–4.
26. Goldhaber SZ. Thrombolysis for pulmonary embolism. N Engl J Med 2002; 347(15):1131–2.
27. Kearon C, Akl EA, Ornelas J, et al. Antithrombotic therapy for VTE disease: CHEST guideline and expert panel report. Chest 2016;149(2):315–52.
28. Kearon C, Akl EA, Comerota AJ, et al. Antithrombotic therapy for VTE disease: antithrombotic therapy and prevention of thrombosis, 9th ed: American College of Chest Physicians evidence-based clinical practice guidelines. Chest 2012; 141(2 Suppl):e419S–96S.
29. Bradford MA, Lindenauer PK, Walkey AJ. Practice patterns and complication rates of thrombolysis for pulmonary embolism. J Thromb Thrombolysis 2016; 42(3):313–21.
30. Dotter CT, Seaman AJ, Rösch J, et al. Streptokinase and heparin in the treatment of pulmonary embolism: a randomized comparison. Vasc Surg 1979;13(1):42–52.
31. Ly B, Arnesen H, Eie H, et al. A controlled clinical trial of streptokinase and heparin in the treatment of major pulmonary embolism. Acta Med Scand 1978;203(6): 465–70.
32. Jerjes-Sanchez C, Ramirez-Rivera A, de Lourdes Garcia M, et al. Streptokinase and heparin versus heparin alone in massive pulmonary embolism: a randomized controlled trial. J Thromb Thrombolysis 1995;2(3):227–9.

33. Wan S, Quinlan DJ, Agnelli G, et al. Thrombolysis compared with heparin for the initial treatment of pulmonary embolism: a meta-analysis of the randomized controlled trials. Circulation 2004;110(6):744–9.

34. Stein PD, Matta F. Thrombolytic therapy in unstable patients with acute pulmonary embolism: saves lives but underused. Am J Med 2012;125(5):465–70.

35. Thrombosis Canada. Pulmonary embolism: diagnosis and management 2018. Available at: http://thrombosiscanada.ca/wp-content/uploads/2018/07/Pulmonary-Embolism-Treatment-2018June15.pdf. Accessed August 01,2019.

36. Goldhaber SZ, Haire WD, Feldstein ML, et al. Alteplase versus heparin in acute pulmonary embolism: randomised trial assessing right-ventricular function and pulmonary perfusion. Lancet 1993;341(8844):507–11.

37. Konstantinides S, Geibel A, Heusel G, et al. Management strategies and prognosis of pulmonary embolism-3 trial investigators. Heparin plus alteplase compared with heparin alone in patients with submassive pulmonary embolism. N Engl J Med 2002;347(15):1143–50.

38. Fasullo S, Scalzo S, Maringhini G, et al. Six-month echocardiographic study in patients with submassive pulmonary embolism and right ventricle dysfunction: comparison of thrombolysis with heparin. Am J Med Sci 2011;341(1):33–9.

39. Kline JA, Nordenholz KE, Courtney DM, et al. Treatment of submassive pulmonary embolism with tenecteplase or placebo: cardiopulmonary outcomes at 3 months: multicenter double-blind, placebo-controlled randomized trial. J Thromb Haemost 2014;12(4):459–68.

40. Meyer G, Vicaut E, Danays T, et al. Fibrinolysis for patients with intermediate-risk pulmonary embolism. N Engl J Med 2014;370(15):1402–11.

41. Kucher N, Boekstegers P, Muller OJ, et al. Randomized, controlled trial of ultrasound-assisted catheter-directed thrombolysis for acute intermediate-risk pulmonary embolism. Circulation 2014;129(4):479–86.

42. Bajaj NS, Kalra R, Arora P, et al. Catheter-directed treatment for acute pulmonary embolism: systematic review and single-arm meta-analyses. Int J Cardiol 2016; 225:128–39.

43. Mostafa A, Briasoulis A, Telila T, et al. Treatment of massive or submassive acute pulmonary embolism with catheter-directed thrombolysis. Am J Cardiol 2016; 117(6):1014–20.

44. Becattini C, Vedovati MC, Agnelli G. Prognostic value of troponins in acute pulmonary embolism: a meta-analysis. Circulation 2007;116(4):427–33.

45. Sanchez O, Trinquart L, Colombet I, et al. Prognostic value of right ventricular dysfunction in patients with haemodynamically stable pulmonary embolism: a systematic review. Eur Heart J 2008;29(12):1569–77.

46. Musani MH. Asymptomatic saddle pulmonary embolism: case report and literature review. Clin Appl Thromb Hemost 2011;17(4):337–9.

47. Activase (alteplase): highlights of prescribing information. 2015. Available at: https://www.accessdata.fda.gov/drugsatfda_docs/label/2015/103172s5203lbl.pdf. Accessed August 1, 2019.

48. Levine M, Hirsh J, Weitz J, et al. A randomized trial of a single bolus dosage regimen of recombinant tissue plasminogen activator in patients with acute pulmonary embolism. Chest 1990;98(6):1473–9.

49. Goldhaber SZ, Agnelli G, Levine MN. Reduced dose bolus alteplase vs conventional alteplase infusion for pulmonary embolism thrombolysis. an international multicenter randomized trial. the bolus alteplase pulmonary embolism group. Chest 1994;106(3):718–24.

50. Sors H, Pacouret G, Azarian R, et al. Hemodynamic effects of bolus vs 2-h infusion of alteplase in acute massive pulmonary embolism. A randomized controlled multicenter trial. Chest 1994;106(3):712–7.
51. Wang C, Zhai Z, Yang Y, et al. Efficacy and safety of low dose recombinant tissue-type plasminogen activator for the treatment of acute pulmonary thromboembolism: a randomized, multicenter, controlled trial. Chest 2010;137(2):254–62.
52. Zhang Z, Zhai ZG, Liang LR, et al. Lower dosage of recombinant tissue-type plasminogen activator (rt-PA) in the treatment of acute pulmonary embolism: a systematic review and meta-analysis. Thromb Res 2014;133(3):357–63.
53. Wang TF, Squizzato A, Dentali F, et al. The role of thrombolytic therapy in pulmonary embolism. Blood 2015;125(14):2191–9.
54. Mikkola KM, Patel SR, Parker JA, et al. Increasing age is a major risk factor for hemorrhagic complications after pulmonary embolism thrombolysis. Am Heart J 1997;134(1):69–72.
55. Daniels LB, Parker JA, Patel SR, et al. Relation of duration of symptoms with response to thrombolytic therapy in pulmonary embolism. Am J Cardiol 1997; 80(2):184–8.
56. Dudzinski DM, Piazza G. Multidisciplinary pulmonary embolism response teams. Circulation 2016;133(1):98–103.
57. Agnelli G, Parise P. Bolus thrombolysis in venous thromboembolism. Chest 1992; 101(4 Suppl):172S–82S.

Interventional Radiology Therapy
Inferior Vena Cava Filter and Catheter-based Therapies

David M. Ruohoniemi, BS, Akhilesh K. Sista, MD*

KEYWORDS

- Catheter-directed therapy • Catheter-directed thrombolysis • Inferior vena cava filter

KEY POINTS

- Indications and use of catheter-directed therapy (CDT) and inferior vena cava filters (IVCFs) for pulmonary embolism (PE) are evolving as new evidence becomes available. Society guidelines differ regarding appropriate use.
- CDT has potential benefits compared with systemic thrombolysis, including rapid onset of action, lower risk of bleeding, fewer bleeding-related contraindications, and long-term reductions in pulmonary pressures. Mechanical thrombectomy is indicated in massive PE, whereas catheter thrombolysis is traditionally preferred in select patients with high-risk submassive PE. New aspiration systems are emerging with preliminary evidence supporting their safety and efficacy for the treatment of submassive PE.
- IVCFs are indicated for high-risk patients with contraindications to anticoagulation or who have failed anticoagulation. Patients who have low cardiopulmonary reserve, including those with massive PE, are also likely to benefit. There is a paucity of evidence supporting the routine use of IVCFs in other select populations despite their prevalence.

CATHETER-DIRECTED THERAPIES

Catheter-directed therapy (CDT) for the treatment of acute pulmonary embolism (PE) is based on the stratification systems from the American Heart Association (AHA) and European Society of Cardiology (ESC). These organizations classify PE as massive (high risk), associated with a mortality of 25% to 65%; submassive (intermediate risk), with a mortality of 2% to 9%; and low risk, with a mortality of less than 1%.[1,2] The classification systems are based on the presence of high-risk features, including the presence of hypotension, bradyarrhythmias, right ventricle (RV) dysfunction, and

Department of Radiology, Division of Interventional Radiology, NYU School of Medicine, 660 1st Avenue, Room 318, New York, NY 10016, USA
* Corresponding author.
E-mail address: Akhilesh.Sista@nyulangone.org

Crit Care Clin 36 (2020) 481–495
https://doi.org/10.1016/j.ccc.2020.02.005
0749-0704/20/© 2020 Elsevier Inc. All rights reserved.

evidence of myocardial ischemia. Clinical scoring systems such as the Simplified Pulmonary Embolism Severity Index (sPESI), derived from the original PESI scoring system, have been incorporated into the stratification systems.[3,4] The ESC subdivides submassive PE into intermediate-high and intermediate-low risk groups based on the presence of both RV dysfunction and increased cardiac troponin levels (intermediate-high) or the presence of 1 or neither of these risk factors (intermediate-low).

Given the low risk of mortality and lack of ventricular dysfunction associated with low-risk PE, these patients can be managed with therapeutic anticoagulation.[5] In contrast, the high mortalities associated with massive PE necessitate more aggressive therapy, including systemic thrombolysis with consideration of CDT or surgical embolectomy.[1,2,5,6] For massive PE, both the AHA and ESC recommend that CDT and surgical embolectomy be considered if there is a contraindication to systemic thrombolysis or for patients who remain hemodynamically unstable. There is considerable uncertainty surrounding the optimal treatment of submassive PE because the benefits of escalation to invasive therapy must be weighed against the risk of intervention, whereas the benefits of systemic thrombolysis must be weighed against the risk of major bleeding. For these patients, the AHA recommends consideration of systemic thrombolysis, CDT, and surgical embolectomy in those with clinical evidence of adverse prognosis. The ESC recommends anticoagulation alone for intermediate-risk to low-risk patients and recommends careful monitoring of intermediate-risk to high-risk patients with PE and consideration of reperfusion for those who are at risk for decompensation. In the ESC treatment algorithm, CDT and surgical embolectomy are considered in lieu of systemic thrombolysis in those with a high bleeding risk (**Table 1**).[2,7]

Catheter-Directed Therapy Overview

CDT involves percutaneous venous access, most commonly through the right common femoral vein, followed by catheterization of the pulmonary artery.[8] Catheterization allows direct measurement of pulmonary arterial, right atrial, and right ventricular pressures. Pulmonary arteriography additionally assesses flow, although it is frequently unnecessary given the accuracy and prevalence of multidetector computed tomography (CT) angiography. The catheter is then advanced to the occlusive thrombus, which is ideally centrally located (main or lobar distribution). The specific catheter-based therapy is initiated depending on the clinical indication. CDT is a broad term that includes endovascular aspiration, fragmentation, and/or dissolution of PEs.[7] Depending on the clinical indication and selected therapy, the patient may return to the angiography suite for completion angiography and pressure reassessment. In many clinical settings, the catheter may be removed at the bedside.

Advantages of Catheter-Directed Therapy

In acute PE, hemodynamic abnormalities caused by acute pulmonary arterial obstruction and vasoconstriction lead to increased mean pulmonary artery pressure (mPAP). Increased mPAP leads to an overloaded RV with subsequent compensatory dilatation and hypokinesis. Displacement of the interventricular septum, as shown by an increased RV/left ventricle (LV) ratio, reduces LV filling and further contributes to ischemia and hypotension.[9] Early studies recognized that the multifactorial derangements during PE are more rapidly addressed by thrombolytic therapy compared with the delayed onset of action of anticoagulation.[10] Despite more rapid action than anticoagulation alone, systemic thrombolysis still requires hours to reach peak effect.[5] The goal of CDT is to rapidly restore pulmonary blood flow and reverse the multifactorial derangements induced by PE.

Table 1
Major society recommendations for the use of catheter-directed therapies

Society	Recommendation
AHA	Catheter embolectomy and fragmentation (or surgical embolectomy):
	Is reasonable for patients with massive PE and contraindications to fibrinolysis
	Is reasonable for patients with massive PE who remain unstable after receiving fibrinolysis
	May be considered for patients with submassive PE with evidence of adverse prognosis
	Is not recommended for patients with low-risk PE or submassive PE without adverse prognosis
ESC	Percutaneous catheter-directed treatment:
	Should be considered for patients with high-risk PE who fail thrombolysis or who have contraindications to thrombolysis
	Should be considered as an alternative rescue thrombolytic therapy for those with intermediate-risk or low-risk PE with hemodynamic deterioration on anticoagulation
ACCP	Catheter-assisted thrombus removal is suggested for patients with acute PE associated with hypotension who have a high bleeding risk, failed systemic thrombolysis, or shock that is likely to cause death before systemic thrombolysis can take effect (hours)
	Remarks that patients who have a higher bleeding risk with systemic thrombolytic therapy treated at centers with access to CDT are likely to choose CDT
SIR	CDT or thrombolysis is an acceptable treatment option for carefully selected patients with proximal massive PE
	Encourages investigative use of CDT and new endovascular techniques in prospective clinical trials, particularly in acute submassive PE

Abbreviations: ACCP, American College of Chest Physicians; SIR, Society of Interventional Radiology.

Beyond the rapid relief of obstruction, CDT has several potential benefits compared with systemic thrombolysis. Depending on the catheter-based intervention, clot removal can be achieved with either locally delivered reduced-dose thrombolytics (tissue plasminogen activator [tPA] or urokinase) or no thrombolytics. Many patients with massive or submassive PE are unable to receive full-dose thrombolytics because of a variety of relative and absolute contraindications, most notably recent surgery, closed-head trauma, prior intracranial hemorrhage, and known structural or malignant cerebrovascular disease.[1,5] Even after careful patient selection, there are considerably high rates of major bleeding, including 20% in the ICOPER (International Cooperative Pulmonary Embolism Registry) and 9.2% in a 2014 meta-analysis of 16 trials comprising 2115 patients.[11,12]

The most commonly used Food and Drug Administration (FDA)–approved systemic thrombolysis regimen for massive PE is 100 mg of alteplase (recombinant tPA) infused through a peripheral access site over a 2-hour period.[1] Although a variety of regimens have been used in landmark studies, systemic thrombolysis has consistently been shown to increase the risk of major bleeding relative to anticoagulation alone.[12–15] Increased bleeding risk may be acceptable in patients with massive PE where systemic thrombolysis has been shown to improve mortality.[12,13] However, the risk/benefit ratio is unclear in submassive PE, where the risk of major and intracerebral bleeding must be weighed against the unclear mortality benefit.[12,13] Therefore, CDT may be beneficial in patients with contraindications to systemic thrombolysis and those with submassive PE.

Another potential benefit of CDT is the possibility of reducing the incidence of pulmonary hypertension, as shown by postpulmonary emboli syndrome and chronic thromboembolic pulmonary hypertension (CTEPH). Anticoagulation alone has a longer time to onset and does not actively dissolve thrombus, leading to retained thrombus that can increase pulmonary pressures. An estimated 3.8% of patients with acute PE develop CTEPH, which may occur despite adequate treatment.[16,17] Roughly 25% of patients were found to have residual pulmonary hypertension at 6 months after submassive PE despite anticoagulation.[18] Evidence from the TOPCOAT (Tenecteplase or Placebo: Cardiopulmonary Outcomes at Three months) and MOPETT (Moderate pulmonary embolism treated with thrombolysis) studies, among others, suggests that systemic thrombolysis may lead to sustained improvements in RV function and pulmonary artery pressure.[19–21] CDT has been shown to reduce the incidence of postthrombotic syndrome in the treatment of deep venous thrombosis (DVT) at 5 years.[22] Taken together, there is considerable interest that CDT may provide similar long-term benefits in the reduction of pulmonary hypertension.

Interventional Perspective on Catheter-Directed Therapy

Based on these advantages and the following data, there is a potential role for CDT in both massive and submassive PE. The Society of Interventional Radiology (SIR) 2018 position statement on CDT for acute PE supports the use of CDT in carefully selected patients with proximal massive PE, especially those rapidly deteriorating despite systemic thrombolysis (see **Table 1**).[23] The SIR recognizes that there are currently insufficient data to recommend routine use of CDT for submassive PE. However, the committee acknowledges that CDT has many advantages compared with other treatment modalities. The SIR recommends that patients with submassive PE be monitored closely for clinical deterioration that should trigger activation of a multidisciplinary team to consider the need for treatment escalation.

Mechanical devices

Overview of mechanical devices Massive PE with hemodynamic shock or decompensation requires rapid thrombus removal, which can be achieved with mechanical techniques, including fragmentation and aspiration. Fragmentation is most often achieved with widely available rotatable pigtail catheters that mechanically disperse the embolus.[24,25] Fragmentation remains the most commonly implemented approach for massive PE and may be used with or without adjunctive lysis, aspiration, and balloon angioplasty.

The relationship between fragmentation and local infusion of lytic medication is not well understood. In 1 study, fragmentation alone caused distal embolization of thrombus with significant increase of mPAP in 7 out of 25 (28%) patients. Increased mPAP improved with subsequent local fibrinolysis and clot aspiration.[26] In contrast, fragmentation increases the surface area of thrombus exposed to locally delivered fibrinolytic drug. A simulated flow study showed that locally delivered fibrinolytics without fragmentation may be less effective because of rapid washout into the nonoccluded pulmonary arteries.[27] Similar to fragmentation, aspiration thrombectomy can be achieved with many widely available 8-Fr end-hole catheters, although new aspiration-specific catheter systems are emerging.

Evidence for mechanical devices There remains a paucity of high-level evidence supporting the use of CDT in massive PE despite theoretic advantages. In a 2009 systematic review and meta-analysis of CDT for massive PE conducted by Kuo and colleagues,[28] most interventions (69%) were accomplished with fragmentation alone

(53%) or in combination with other maneuvers (16%). Although other treatment modalities were included in the investigators' definition of modern CDT (low-profile device ≤10-Fr, mechanical fragmentation and/or aspiration, and intraclot fibrinolytic infusion), the pooled clinical success rate (86.5%) in this cohort supports the use of mechanical fragmentation (**Table 2**). Of note, 95% (546 out of 571) of the patients were treated with CDT as the first adjunct to heparin and did not receive systemic thrombolysis before catheterization. The investigators concluded that modern CDT is relatively safe and effective for treatment of acute massive PE.[28]

As mentioned, the 2009 landmark meta-analysis included a variety of devices. However, of particular interest is the AngioJet rheolytic device (Boston Scientific; Marlborough, MA). This device uses saline jets to create a low-pressure zone, thus generating a vacuum effect. The meta-analysis from Kuo and colleagues[28] found a low pooled risk of minor (7.9%) and major (2.4%) procedural complications. High complication rates from the 68 patients treated with the AngioJet device were seen, including a 40% minor complication rate, 28% major complication rate, and 5 procedure-related deaths. The FDA subsequently issued a black box warning for use in PE. In all, traditional mechanical devices have shown good clinical success rates and low complication rates in the treatment of massive PE but were not extensively studied in the treatment of submassive PE.

Catheter-directed thrombolysis

Overview of catheter-directed thrombolysis Catheter-directed thrombolysis, also known as catheter-directed fibrinolysis, delivers reduced-dose fibrinolytics through a multisidehole catheter with or without adjunctive ultrasonic assistance. Unlike systemic thrombolysis, which is most often achieved with 100 mg of tPA over a 2-hour infusion, catheter-directed thrombolysis can deliver higher drug concentrations within the thrombus at a much lower systemic dose.[29,30] Once the catheter is positioned within the thrombus, a bolus of tPA (approximately 5 mg) may be delivered, followed by continuous infusion. Up to 2 infusion catheters may be placed and tPA infused at a rate of 0.5 to 1 mg/h per catheter for 12 to 24 hours.[31] A total dose of 15 to 30 mg of tPA is typically used.

Although mechanical approaches are often favored for massive PE where immediate debulking is required to avoid cardiovascular collapse, there is a risk of distal embolization and worsening pulmonary hypertension.[27] Therefore, catheter-directed thrombolysis has become standard practice for catheter-based treatment of submassive PE. As discussed previously, treatment algorithms are complex and depend on local expertise and available therapies. As a result, there is considerable crossover. Mechanical techniques have been studied in submassive PE, and catheter-directed thrombolysis has been used in massive PE.

Evidence for catheter-directed thrombolysis Despite the consensus that CDT has a role in massive PE, the evidence for CDT in submassive PE remains elusive.[12,23,32] There is a lack of randomized controlled trials that provide compelling evidence for the use of catheter-directed rather than systemic thrombolysis. Three prospective studies have collectively shown that thrombolysis dissolves PEs, restores RV function, and improves pulmonary blood flow. In these studies, catheter-directed thrombolysis has been associated with low major and intracranial bleeding rates (see **Table 2**).

The ULTIMA (Ultrasound Assisted Thrombolysis of Pulmonary Embolism) and SEATTLE II (EkoSonic Endovascular System and Activase for Treatment of Acute Pulmonary Embolism) trials provide evidence for the EkoSonic Endovascular System (Ekos/BTG; Bothell, WA). The EkoSonic catheter produces high-frequency ultrasonic

Table 2
Summary of data from recent clinical trials of catheter-directed therapy for acute pulmonary embolism

Technique	Study	Design	Notable Findings
Fragmentation	Kuo et al,[28] 2009	Systematic review and meta-analysis of modern CDT for massive PE. Included 549 patients from 35 studies	Pooled clinical success rate of 86.5%. CDT as first adjunct to heparin in 95% of patients. Low pooled minor (7.9%) and major (2.4%) complication rate
Thrombolysis	ULTIMA, 2014	Randomized 59 patients with submassive PE to USAT plus anticoagulation or anticoagulation alone	USAT was superior to anticoagulation alone in reversing RV dilatation at 24 h (0.30 vs 0.03, $P<.001$). No increase in bleeding complications, including no major bleeds in either group
	PERFECT, 2015	Prospectively enrolled 101 consecutive patients (28 massive, 73 submassive) who received CDT for acute PE	Good clinical success rate for massive (85.7%) and submassive (97.3%) PE. Improvement in mPAP and right heart strain ($P<.001$). No procedure-related complications or major bleeds
	SEATTLE II, 2015	Prospectively enrolled 150 patients (31 massive, 119 submassive) treated with USAT	Reductions in RV/LV ratio (-0.42, $P<.0001$) and mPAP (51.4 vs 36.9, $P<.0001$) at 48 h. One severe bleed and 16 moderate bleeding events. No intracranial hemorrhage
	OPTALYSE PE, 2018	Randomized 100 patients treated with USAT to 4 different tPA dosing regimens	Shorter delivery duration and lower-dose tPA was associated with improved RV function ($P = .0001$). Four major bleeds (4%) with 1 procedure-related intracranial hemorrhage
Aspiration	FLARE	Prospectively enrolled 106 patients with submassive PE treated with mechanical thrombectomy	Reduction in RV/LV ratio (-0.38, $P<.0001$) and 43 patients (41.3%) did not require ICU stay. Four patients (3.8%) with major adverse events, 1 experienced major bleeding

Abbreviations: FLARE; FlowTriever Pulmonary Embolectomy Clinical Study; ICU, intensive care unit; PERFECT, Pulmonary Embolism Response to Fragmentation, Embolectomy, and Catheter Thrombolysis; SEATTLE, EkoSonic Endovascular System and Activase for Treatment of Acute Pulmonary Embolism; ULTIMA, Ultrasound Assisted Thrombolysis of Pulmonary Embolism; USAT, ultrasonography-assisted thrombolysis.

waves to facilitate clot disintegration as the fibrinolytic drug is infused, termed ultrasonography-assisted catheter-directed thrombolysis (USAT). The device received FDA approval in 2014 following results of the ULTIMA and SEATTLE II studies.

The randomized ULTIMA study (2014) enrolled 59 patients with acute submassive PE to treatment with USAT plus heparin or heparin alone. There was a significant difference in the reduction in the RV/LV ratio between groups (0.30 vs 0.03, $P<.001$) at 24 hours.[33] The single-arm SEATTLE II registry enrolled both patients with submassive PE (119) and massive PE (31) treated with USAT. At 48 hours, there was a reduction in the mean RV/LV ratio (-0.42, $P<.0001$) and mPAP (51.4 vs 36.9 mm Hg, $P<.0001$).[34] Of the combined 180 patients treated with USAT in these trials, there was only 1 severe bleed (groin hematoma with transient hypotension) and no intracranial hemorrhages. More recently, the OPTALYSE (A Randomized Trial of the Optimum Duration of Acoustic Pulse Thrombolysis Procedure in Acute Intermediate-Risk Pulmonary Embolism) PE trial (2018) investigated the optimal dose and delivery duration of USAT and found similar changes in the RV/LV ratio between the lowest dosing regimen (4 mg/lung/2 h) compared with higher dosing regimens (up to 12 mg/lung/ 6 h).[35] It is difficult to know whether these changes are a result of USAT given that there was no control group.

In addition, the PERFECT (Pulmonary Embolism Response to Fragmentation, Embolectomy, and Catheter Thrombolysis) registry enrolled patients with submassive (73) or massive (28) PE who were treated with CDT. Similar to the ULTIMA and SEATTLE II studies, there was a reduction in the mPAP (51.2 vs 37.2 mm Hg, $P<.0001$) and no major hemorrhages or hemorrhagic stroke.[36] The investigators concluded that CDT is safe and effective in the treatment of both massive and submassive PE. As a whole, these studies provide evidence that catheter-directed thrombolysis is safe and effective at improving short-term RV function, primarily in patients with submassive PE (see **Table 2**).

Emerging aspiration devices

FlowTriever The FlowTriever System (Inari Medical; Irvine, CA) received FDA 510(k) approval for the treatment of PE in 2018. It is currently the only mechanical thrombectomy device indicated for PE. The device consists of a 20-Fr aspiration guide catheter (AGC, Triever20) and a FlowTriever Catheter that is delivered through the AGC and contains 3 self-expanding nitinol mesh disks.[37] Aspiration is achieved by generating negative pressure through a 50-cm^3 syringe.[38] Aspiration may be performed through the AGC alone or clot may be captured by the nitinol disks and withdrawn into the AGC before aspiration. An example case is shown in **Fig. 1**.

Unlike the previously discussed fragmentation and aspiration devices, the FlowTriever was not included in the 2009 Kuo and colleagues[28] meta-analysis. However, the recently published FlowTriever Pulmonary Embolectomy Clinical Study (FLARE) provides evidence for patients with submassive PE.[37] This single-arm, prospective, multi-institutional study enrolled 106 patients from 18 US sites with acute submassive PE. The investigators showed significant reduction in the RV/LV ratio (-0.38, 25%, $P<.0001$) following percutaneous mechanical thrombectomy. In addition, there was a low major adverse event rate (3.8%) within 48 hours of the procedure, low rate of major bleeding (1.0%), and a significant minority of patients did not require admission to the intensive care unit (41.3%, see **Table 2**). Of note, the study excluded patients with contraindications to anticoagulation therapy. The study was limited by a lack of a comparison group, short-term follow-up (30 days), and indirect efficacy measures. Based on these results, the investigators concluded that the FlowTriever is safe and effective for submassive PE, with potential benefits including immediate thrombus

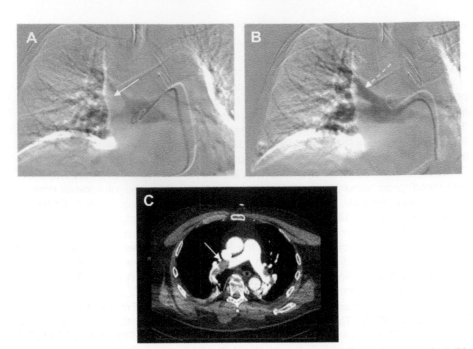

Fig. 1. Representative case of percutaneous mechanical thrombectomy (FlowTriever). A 54-year-old man developed massive PE after resection of a glioblastoma. (*A*) Preintervention right pulmonary angiogram shows thrombus (*arrow*) at the bifurcation of the right main pulmonary artery (mPAP, 35 mm Hg). (*B*) Postintervention angiogram shows improved perfusion (*dashed arrow*) in the area of interest (mPAP, 26 mm Hg). (*C*) Preintervention CT angiogram reveals the extent of thrombus within proximal right pulmonary artery (*solid arrow*).

removal, absence of thrombolytic complications, and a reduced need for postprocedure care.[37]

Publication of the FLARE study was followed by a real-world single-center retrospective experience that included 46 patients (8 massive, 38 submassive) treated with the FlowTriever device.[38] All patients treated with the FlowTriever were included, comprising patients with contraindications to thrombolysis that likely would have been excluded from the FLARE study. Wible and colleagues[38] found a significant reduction in mPAP in both the massive (*P*<.05) and submassive (*P*<.001) groups, with a reduction in intraprocedural mPAP in 37 out of 42 patients (88%). Similar to the FLARE study, there were few major adverse events (4.6%) and no procedure-related deaths at 30 days.

Although these studies add to the growing literature surrounding emerging aspiration thrombectomy devices, questions remain. Both studies reported a case of massive hemoptysis, likely from tracking a large 20-Fr catheter across delicate structures. Neither study reported long-term outcomes or defined the optimal use of the device (ie, number of passes, role for adjunctive fibrinolytics).[39] To address these deficiencies, an observational registry has begun enrollment with a target of 500 patients and a planned 6-month follow-up (FLASH [FlowTriever All-Comer Registry for Patient Safety and Hemodynamics], Clinical Trials Identifier NCT03761173). The registry will help evaluate safety and efficacy in a real-world population, including both massive and submassive PE.

Indigo and AngioVac The findings of the FLARE study are the first in a series of expected publications for several emerging aspiration devices. Other devices include the Indigo Mechanical Thrombectomy System (Penumbra; Alameda, CA) and the AngioVac (AngioDynamics; Latham, NY). The Indigo system provides continuous suction powered by an engine that delivers negative pressure. Early studies of the Indigo system have shown promise in the treatment of acute massive and submassive PE in both prospective registries and retrospective analyses.[40–42] As with other studies, the results are limited by indirect measures of success, small sample sizes, and by short follow-up times. The ongoing EXTRACT-PE (Evaluating the Safety and Efficacy of the Indigo Aspiration System in Acute Pulmonary Embolism) study (Clinical Trials Identifier NCT03218566) is scheduled to complete enrollment of 119 patients in September 2019 and will provide more robust data, including 48-hour and 30-day outcomes. The AngioVac is a venovenous bypass system that is FDA approved for the removal of thrombus during extracorporeal bypass. Early experiences revealed moderate success rates but concerns were raised regarding technical aspects, safety, and high cost.[43,44] Real-world results from the ongoing RAPID (Registry of Angiovac Procedures in Detail Outcomes Database) registry may help clarify the role of the AngioVac device in PE management.

Summary of catheter-directed therapy for pulmonary embolism CDT has potential benefits compared with systemic thrombolysis, including rapid onset, access to the pulmonary vasculature, lack of systemic fibrinolysis (ie, lower bleeding risk), fewer bleeding-related contraindications, and perhaps long-term benefits. Major societies recognize the role of CDT for massive PE, particularly in patients with contraindications to systemic fibrinolysis or who remain unstable.[1,2,5,23] When indicated, mechanical thrombectomy is preferred for massive PE to avoid acute cardiovascular collapse. For submassive PE, there is ongoing debate regarding the role of CDT because of a lack of high-quality evidence. Traditionally, catheter-directed thrombolysis was preferred for submassive PE because it was perceived to have lower risk of worsening pulmonary hypertension. However, new studies support the use of emerging aspiration devices in the treatment of submassive PE.

INFERIOR VENA CAVA FILTERS
Indications

There is debate regarding the appropriate clinical indications for inferior vena cava filter (IVCF) placement. Filters, both permanent and retrievable (optional), are most commonly placed in an infrarenal location with the goal of preventing PE in high-risk patients. IVCF use gained popularity in the 1990s and increased rapidly into the early 2000s.[45,46] The increase came despite concerns that filters may not adequately prevent recurrent PE or improve mortality.[47,48]

The results of the PREPIC 2 (Prevention du Risque d'Embolie Pulmonaire par Interruption Cave 2) study revealed that IVCF placement in addition to anticoagulation did not decrease recurrent PE at 3 months for patients with acute PE and a high risk of recurrence.[49] Furthermore, a 2017 systematic review and meta-analysis revealed that IVCFs may decrease the risk of recurrent PE without affecting overall mortality.[50] The study also revealed that there is a dearth of high-quality evidence for IVCF placement. As a result, filter placement has declined over the last decade.[51,52] The lack of data coupled with low retrieval rates and the risks associated with both IVCF placement and prolonged dwelling (perforation, thrombosis, migration, tilt) prompted the FDA to issue a 2010 advisory recommending early filter removal.[53,54]

Controversy

The steady increase in IVCF placement was caused, in part, by expanding indications despite low-quality evidence. As a result, society guidelines regarding the appropriate use of IVCFs are not uniform (**Table 3**).[1,2,5,55] There is consensus that IVCFs are indicated in patients following acute venous thromboembolism who have contraindications to anticoagulation and those who fail anticoagulation.[1,2,5,55,56] The use of IVCFs for high-risk patients with poor cardiopulmonary reserve is also widely accepted despite poor prospective data.

Guidelines differ on indications for filter placement, including prophylactic indications and free-floating iliofemoral or inferior vena cava thrombus. The SIR and American College of Radiology (ACR) advocate more widely applicable criteria compared with the AHA and ESC (see **Table 3**). Prophylactic use of filters in high-risk patients (trauma, spinal surgery, prolonged immobilization) is particularly controversial. There is conflicting evidence regarding the use of IVCF in these patients.[57–61] Similarly, the evidence for IVCF for free-floating DVT is lacking. Early studies suggest that these patients are high risk for embolic events, but prospective evidence is lacking.[62,63]

Inferior Vena Cava Filters in Pulmonary Embolism

Two indications of particular interest in endovascular PE management are the use of filters for hemodynamically unstable patients (massive PE) with residual thrombus and those undergoing treatment, particularly CDT. Patients with massive PE are unstable by definition with low cardiopulmonary reserve, putting them at high risk for hemodynamic compromise caused by further embolic events. National registry data have shown that patients with unstable PE benefitted from IVCF, whether or not they received thrombolysis.[11,64,65] As a result, there is general agreement that this population may benefit from IVCF placement.[1,5,55,56]

In contrast, routine placement of IVCFs for submassive PE is not recommended if the patient can be anticoagulated because of associated risks and a lack of high-level evidence.[49,66] There is no evidence regarding the placement of IVCFs during CDT for submassive PE. Despite this, filters are occasionally placed, including in 16% of patients in the SEATTLE II study.[34] At our institution, IVCFs are not placed for submassive PE at the time of CDT, in part because of the risk of maneuvering catheters and sheaths past the filter. Of note, there is considerable debate regarding the role of IVCF placement before CDT for DVT. Reported rates of PE following CDT for DVT vary widely.[67–69] A recent nationwide observational study suggests that, despite the frequent use of IVCFs in this patient population (34%), it does not decrease in-hospital mortality but increases charges and length of stay.[70]

Table 3
Select indications for inferior vena cava filter placement as supported by major society guidelines

Indications	Supported by Society Guidelines
Acute PE and absolute contraindication to thrombolysis	AHA, ESC, ACCP, SIR
Recurrent acute PE despite therapeutic anticoagulation	AHA, ESC, SIR
Acute PE and very low cardiopulmonary reserve	AHA, ACCP, SIR
Free-floating iliofemoral or inferior vena cava thrombus, prophylaxis (severe trauma, closed-head injury, spinal cord injury, multiple fractures, high risk)	SIR

Summary of Inferior Vena Cava Filters

Understanding of IVCFs has evolved as early enthusiasm has been tempered by larger recent studies. Filters definitively play a role in patients with contraindications or who fail anticoagulation. However, high-quality evidence for the increased use and indications for IVCFs is lacking. Filters have a role in patients with massive PE and patients with poor cardiopulmonary reserve. However, further studies are required to define their role in the treatment of submassive PE, high-risk surgical patients, and those undergoing CDT for proximal DVT.

SUMMARY

Endovascular therapy for the treatment and prophylaxis of PE is evolving as higher-quality evidence becomes available. Select patients with massive and submassive PE may benefit from CDT. Both catheter-directed thrombolysis and catheter-based embolectomy have shown good short-term efficacy based on surrogate outcomes with low bleeding rates. Future randomized trials are needed to assess short-term and long-term clinical outcomes and identify patients who will benefit most. IVCF use is declining after years of steady growth as expanding indications are called into question. Although there are a few clear indications, aligning society recommendations will depend on the emergence of randomized studies.

DISCLOSURE

A.K. Sista: research support from Penumbra, Inc.

REFERENCES

1. Jaff MR, McMurtry MS, Archer SL, et al. Management of massive and submassive pulmonary embolism, iliofemoral deep vein thrombosis, and chronic thromboembolic pulmonary hypertension. Circulation 2011;123(16):1788–830.
2. Konstantinides SV, Meyer G, Becattini C, et al, for the Task Force for the Diagnosis and Management of Acute Pulmonary Embolism of the European Society of Cardiology (ESC) developed in collaboration with the European Respiratory Society (ERS). 2019 ESC guidelines for the diagnosis and management of acute pulmonary embolism. Eur Respir J 2019. https://doi.org/10.1183/13993003.01647-2019.
3. Wicki J, Perrier A, Perneger TV, et al. Predicting adverse outcome in patients with acute pulmonary embolism: a risk score. Thromb Haemost 2000;84(4):548–52.
4. Jiménez D, Aujesky D, Moores L, et al. Simplification of the pulmonary embolism severity index for prognostication in patients with acute symptomatic pulmonary embolism. Arch Intern Med 2010;170(15):1383–9.
5. Kearon C, Akl EA, Ornelas J, et al. Antithrombotic therapy for VTE disease: CHEST guideline and expert panel report. Chest 2016;149(2):315–52.
6. Jaber WA, Fong PP, Weisz G, et al. Acute pulmonary embolism: with an emphasis on an interventional approach. J Am Coll Cardiol 2016;67(8):991–1002.
7. Javed QA, Sista AK. Endovascular therapy for acute severe pulmonary embolism. Int J Cardiovasc Imaging 2019;35(8):1443–52.
8. Chiarello MA, Sista AK. Catheter-directed thrombolysis for submassive pulmonary embolism. Semin Intervent Radiol 2018;35(2):122–8.
9. Tarbox AK, Swaroop M. Pulmonary embolism. Int J Crit Illn Inj Sci 2013;3(1):69–72.

10. Elliott CG. Pulmonary physiology during pulmonary embolism. Chest 1992;101(4 Suppl):163S–71S.
11. Goldhaber SZ, Visani L, De Rosa M. Acute pulmonary embolism: clinical outcomes in the International Cooperative Pulmonary Embolism Registry (ICOPER). Lancet 1999;353(9162):1386–9.
12. Chatterjee S, Chakraborty A, Weinberg I, et al. Thrombolysis for pulmonary embolism and risk of all-cause mortality, major bleeding, and intracranial hemorrhage: a meta-analysis. JAMA 2014;311(23):2414–21.
13. Marti C, John G, Konstantinides S, et al. Systemic thrombolytic therapy for acute pulmonary embolism: a systematic review and meta-analysis. Eur Heart J 2015; 36(10):605–14.
14. Meyer G, Vicaut E, Danays T, et al. Fibrinolysis for patients with intermediate-risk pulmonary embolism. N Engl J Med 2014;370(15):1402–11.
15. Konstantinides S, Geibel A, Heusel G, et al, for the Management Strategies and Prognosis of Pulmonary Embolism-3 Trial Investigators. Heparin plus alteplase compared with heparin alone in patients with submassive pulmonary embolism. N Engl J Med 2002;347(15):1143–50.
16. Pengo V, Lensing AW, Prins MH, et al. Incidence of chronic thromboembolic pulmonary hypertension after pulmonary embolism. N Engl J Med 2004;350(22): 2257–64.
17. McNeil K, Dunning J. Chronic thromboembolic pulmonary hypertension (CTEPH). Heart 2007;93(9):1152–8.
18. Kline JA, Steuerwald MT, Marchick MR, et al. Prospective evaluation of right ventricular function and functional status 6 months after acute submassive pulmonary embolism. Chest 2009;136(5):1202–10.
19. Kline JA, Nordenholz KE, Courtney DM, et al. Treatment of submassive pulmonary embolism with tenecteplase or placebo: cardiopulmonary outcomes at 3 months: multicenter double-blind, placebo-controlled randomized trial. J Thromb Haemost 2014;12(4):459–68.
20. Sharifi M, Bay C, Skrocki L, et al. Moderate pulmonary embolism treated with thrombolysis (from the "MOPETT" Trial). Am J Cardiol 2013;111(2):273–7.
21. Sharma GV, Folland ED, McIntyre KM, et al. Long-term benefit of thrombolytic therapy in patients with pulmonary embolism. Vasc Med 2000;5(2):91–5.
22. Haig Y, Enden T, Grøtta O, et al, for the CaVenT Study Group. Post-thrombotic syndrome after catheter-directed thrombolysis for deep vein thrombosis (CaVenT): 5-year follow-up results of an open-label, randomised controlled trial. Lancet Haematol 2016;3(2):e64–71.
23. Kuo WT, Sista AK, Faintuch S, et al. Society of Interventional Radiology position statement on catheter-directed therapy for acute pulmonary embolism. J Vasc Interv Radiol 2018;29(3):293–7.
24. Schmitz-Rode T, Janssens U, Schild HH, et al. Fragmentation of massive pulmonary embolism using a pigtail rotation catheter. Chest 1998;114(5):1427–36.
25. Schmitz-Rode T, Janssens U, Duda SH, et al. Massive pulmonary embolism: percutaneous emergency treatment by pigtail rotation catheter. J Am Coll Cardiol 2000;36(2):375–80.
26. Nakazawa K, Tajima H, Murata S, et al. Catheter fragmentation of acute massive pulmonary thromboembolism: distal embolisation and pulmonary arterial pressure elevation. Br J Radiol 2008;81(971):848–54.
27. Schmitz-Rode T, Kilbinger M, Günther RW. Simulated flow pattern in massive pulmonary embolism: significance for selective intrapulmonary thrombolysis. Cardiovasc Intervent Radiol 1998;21(3):199–204.

28. Kuo WT, Gould MK, Louie JD, et al. Catheter-directed therapy for the treatment of massive pulmonary embolism: systematic review and meta-analysis of modern techniques. J Vasc Interv Radiol 2009;20(11):1431–40.
29. Tapson VF. Acute pulmonary embolism. N Engl J Med 2008;358(10):1037–52.
30. Sista AK, Horowitz JM, Goldhaber SZ. Four key questions surrounding thrombolytic therapy for submassive pulmonary embolism. Vasc Med 2016;21(1):47–52.
31. Kuo WT. Endovascular therapy for acute pulmonary embolism. J Vasc Interv Radiol 2012;23(2):167–79.e4.
32. Sista AK, Goldhaber SZ, Vedantham S, et al. Research priorities in submassive pulmonary embolism: proceedings from a multidisciplinary research consensus panel. J Vasc Interv Radiol 2016;27(6):787–94.
33. Kucher N, Boekstegers P, Müller OJ, et al. Randomized, controlled trial of ultrasound-assisted catheter-directed thrombolysis for acute intermediate-risk pulmonary embolism. Circulation 2014;129(4):479–86.
34. Piazza G, Hohlfelder B, Jaff MR, et al, for the SEATTLE II Investigators. A prospective, single-arm, multicenter trial of ultrasound-facilitated, catheter-directed, low-dose fibrinolysis for acute massive and submassive pulmonary embolism: the SEATTLE II Study. JACC Cardiovasc Interv 2015;8(10):1382–92.
35. Tapson VF, Sterling K, Jones N, et al. A randomized trial of the optimum duration of acoustic pulse thrombolysis procedure in acute intermediate-risk pulmonary embolism: the OPTALYSE PE Trial. JACC Cardiovasc Interv 2018;11(14): 1401–10.
36. Kuo WT, Banerjee A, Kim PS, et al. Pulmonary embolism Response to fragmentation, embolectomy, and catheter thrombolysis (PERFECT): initial results from a prospective multicenter registry. Chest 2015;148(3):667–73.
37. Tu T, Toma C, Tapson VF, et al, for the FLARE Investigators. A prospective, single-arm, multicenter trial of catheter-directed mechanical thrombectomy for intermediate-risk acute pulmonary embolism: the FLARE Study. JACC Cardiovasc Interv 2019;12(9):859–69.
38. Wible BC, Buckley JR, Cho KH, et al. Safety and efficacy of acute pulmonary embolism treated via large-bore aspiration mechanical thrombectomy using the Inari FlowTriever device. J Vasc Interv Radiol 2019;30(9):1370–5.
39. Sista AK. Aspiration thrombectomy for severe pulmonary embolism using the FlowTriever device: the good, the bad, and the unknown. J Vasc Interv Radiol 2019;30(9):1376–7.
40. Ciampi-Dopazo JJ, Romeu-Prieto JM, Sánchez-Casado M, et al. Aspiration thrombectomy for treatment of acute massive and submassive pulmonary embolism: initial single-center prospective experience. J Vasc Interv Radiol 2018;29(1): 101–6.
41. De Gregorio MA, Guirola JA, Kuo WT, et al. Catheter-directed aspiration thrombectomy and low-dose thrombolysis for patients with acute unstable pulmonary embolism: prospective outcomes from a PE registry. Int J Cardiol 2019;287: 106–10.
42. Al-Hakim R, Bhatt A, Benenati JF. Continuous aspiration mechanical thrombectomy for the management of submassive pulmonary embolism: a single-center experience. J Vasc Interv Radiol 2017;28(10):1348–52.
43. Al-Hakim R, Park J, Bansal A, et al. Early experience with AngioVac aspiration in the pulmonary arteries. J Vasc Interv Radiol 2016;27(5):730–4.
44. Salsamendi J, Doshi M, Bhatia S, et al. Single center experience with the AngioVac aspiration system. Cardiovasc Intervent Radiol 2015;38(4):998–1004.

45. Kuy S, Dua A, Lee CJ, et al. National trends in utilization of inferior vena cava filters in the United States, 2000-2009. J Vasc Surg Venous Lymphat Disord 2014; 2(1):15–20.
46. Duszak R, Parker L, Levin DC, et al. Placement and removal of inferior vena cava filters: national trends in the medicare population. J Am Coll Radiol 2011;8(7): 483–9.
47. PREPIC Study Group. Eight-year follow-up of patients with permanent vena cava filters in the prevention of pulmonary embolism: the PREPIC (Prevention du Risque d'Embolie Pulmonaire par Interruption Cave) randomized study. Circulation 2005;112(3):416–22.
48. Young T, Tang H, Hughes R. Vena caval filters for the prevention of pulmonary embolism. Cochrane Database Syst Rev 2010;(2):CD006212.
49. Mismetti P, Laporte S, Pellerin O, et al, for the PREPIC2 Study Group. Effect of a retrievable inferior vena cava filter plus anticoagulation vs anticoagulation alone on risk of recurrent pulmonary embolism: a randomized clinical trial. JAMA 2015;313(16):1627–35.
50. Bikdeli B, Chatterjee S, Desai NR, et al. Inferior vena cava filters to prevent pulmonary embolism: systematic review and meta-analysis. J Am Coll Cardiol 2017; 70(13):1587–97.
51. Wadhwa V, Trivedi PS, Chatterjee K, et al. Decreasing utilization of inferior vena cava filters in post-FDA warning era: insights from 2005 to 2014 Nationwide Inpatient Sample. J Am Coll Radiol 2017;14(9):1144–50.
52. Morris E, Duszak R, Sista AK, et al. National trends in inferior vena cava filter placement and retrieval procedures in the medicare population over two decades. J Am Coll Radiol 2018;15(8):1080–6.
53. Ahmed O, Wadhwa V, Patel K, et al. Rising retrieval rates of inferior vena cava filters in the United States: insights from the 2012 to 2016 summary medicare claims data. J Am Coll Radiol 2018;15(11):1553–7.
54. Brown JD, Raissi D, Han Q, et al. Vena cava filter retrieval rates and factors associated with retrieval in a large US cohort. J Am Heart Assoc 2017;6(9). https://doi.org/10.1161/JAHA.117.006708.
55. Caplin DM, Nikolic B, Kalva SP, et al, for the Society of Interventional Radiology Standards of Practice Committee. Quality improvement guidelines for the performance of inferior vena cava filter placement for the prevention of pulmonary embolism. J Vasc Interv Radiol 2011;22(11):1499–506.
56. Weinberg I, Kaufman J, Jaff MR. Inferior vena cava filters. JACC Cardiovasc Interv 2013;6(6):539–47.
57. Haut ER, Garcia LJ, Shihab HM, et al. The effectiveness of prophylactic inferior vena cava filters in trauma patients: a systematic review and meta-analysis. JAMA Surg 2014;149(2):194–202.
58. McClendon J, O'shaughnessy BA, Smith TR, et al. Comprehensive assessment of prophylactic preoperative inferior vena cava filters for major spinal reconstruction in adults. Spine 2012;37(13):1122–9.
59. Rutherford RB. Prophylactic indications for vena cava filters: critical appraisal. Semin Vasc Surg 2005;18(3):158–65.
60. Gorman PH, Qadri SFA, Rao-Patel A. Prophylactic inferior vena cava (IVC) filter placement may increase the relative risk of deep venous thrombosis after acute spinal cord injury. J Trauma 2009;66(3):707–12.
61. Ho KM, Rao S, Honeybul S, et al. A multicenter trial of vena cava filters in severely injured patients. N Engl J Med 2019;381(4):328–37.

62. Baldridge ED, Martin MA, Welling RE. Clinical significance of free-floating venous thrombi. J Vasc Surg 1990;11(1):62–7 [discussion: 68–9].
63. Pacouret G, Alison D, Pottier JM, et al. Free-floating thrombus and embolic risk in patients with angiographically confirmed proximal deep venous thrombosis: a prospective study. Arch Intern Med 1997;157(3):305–8.
64. Stein PD, Matta F, Keyes DC, et al. Impact of vena cava filters on in-hospital case fatality rate from pulmonary embolism. Am J Med 2012;125(5):478–84.
65. Stein PD, Matta F. Vena cava filters in unstable elderly patients with acute pulmonary embolism. Am J Med 2014;127(3):222–5.
66. Stein PD, Matta F, Hughes MJ. Inferior vena cava filters in stable patients with acute pulmonary embolism who receive thrombolytic therapy. Am J Med 2018; 131(1):97–9.
67. Mewissen MW, Seabrook GR, Meissner MH, et al. Catheter-directed thrombolysis for lower extremity deep venous thrombosis: report of a national multicenter registry. Radiology 1999;211(1):39–49.
68. Kwon SH, Park SH, Oh JH, et al. Prophylactic placement of an inferior vena cava filter during aspiration thrombectomy for acute deep venous thrombosis of the lower extremity. Vasc Endovascular Surg 2016;50(4):270–6.
69. Jiang J, Tu J, Jia Z, et al. Incidence and outcomes of inferior vena cava filter thrombus during catheter-directed thrombolysis for proximal deep venous thrombosis. Ann Vasc Surg 2017;38:305–9.
70. Akhtar OS, Lakhter V, Zack CJ, et al. Contemporary trends and comparative outcomes with adjunctive inferior vena cava filter placement in patients undergoing catheter-directed thrombolysis for deep vein thrombosis in the United States: insights from the National Inpatient Sample. JACC Cardiovasc Interv 2018;11(14): 1390–7.

Surgical Pulmonary Embolectomy

Dale Shelton Deas, MD, Brent Keeling, MD*

KEYWORDS

- Surgery • Pulmonary embolus • Pulmonary embolectomy

KEY POINTS

- Historically, surgical pulmonary embolectomy was reserved as a salvage procedure for patients who either failed or had an absolute contraindication to thrombolysis.
- The approach to surgical pulmonary embolectomy has been revised since the initial forays by Trendelenburg to incorporate the now ubiquitous cardiopulmonary bypass circuit.
- With the re-emergence of surgery as a safe and viable means of treating patients with large pulmonary emboli, multiple studies have compared surgery to other therapies in the treatment of acute pulmonary embolism.

INTRODUCTION

Surgical pulmonary embolectomy was first described in 1908 by Friedrich Trendelenburg.[1,2] Trendelenburg had great interest in and actively investigated the clinical manifestations of acute pulmonary embolism, including symptoms, physiologic features, and progression of disease from onset to death. As a result of this interest, he then devised an operative plan for massive pulmonary emboli that involved physically removing the embolic debris from the pulmonary artery. Initially, Trendelenburg approached the main pulmonary artery through a left anterior thoracotomy at the second interspace using a transverse incision in conjunction with a perpendicular incision along the left sternal border to expose and divide the second and third ribs anteriorly. The pleura and pericardium were then opened, thus providing optimal exposure. To remove the pulmonary embolism, a 1 cm longitudinal incision was made along the main pulmonary artery extending toward the bifurcation while also occluding the main pulmonary artery and aorta proximal to the incision site using rubber tubing placed in the transverse sinus. This would prevent massive hemorrhage and allow embolic extraction from the pulmonary artery and its branches. Unfortunately, his first attempt at this technique resulted in patient death because of overwhelming hemorrhage.

Division of Cardiothoracic Surgery, Emory University, 550 Peachtree Street, MOT 6th floor, Atlanta, GA 30308, USA
* Corresponding author.
E-mail address: brent.keeling@emory.edu
Twitter: @BrentKeeling (B.K.)

Crit Care Clin 36 (2020) 497–504
https://doi.org/10.1016/j.ccc.2020.02.009
0749-0704/20/© 2020 Elsevier Inc. All rights reserved.

Trendelenburg later attempted this technique with 2 other patients; they both survived the initial procedure but died within 2 days because of right heart failure and hemorrhage. Despite these immediate failures, a plausible technique for surgical intervention had been created, and it eventually became successful. Professor Martin Kirschner, who was a pupil of Trendelenburg, performed the first successful pulmonary embolectomy in 1924 using the technique that Trendelenburg had described. Despite this success, pulmonary embolectomy remained a morbid procedure with high rates of postoperative mortality. John H. Gibbon was particularly discouraged by these outcomes, noting in 1937 that only 9of 142 patients who underwent surgical pulmonary embolectomy survived to discharge from the hospital.[3] This realization led to his interest in and ultimate development of the cardiopulmonary bypass machine, which subsequently changed the landscape of cardiac surgery forever. The first surgical pulmonary embolectomies conducted with cardiopulmonary bypass were performed by Sharp and Cooley in the early 1960s.[4,5] These procedures were successful, and the patients survived to discharge from the hospital. Surgical pulmonary embolectomy, however, was still largely reserved for patients undergoing emergent or salvage procedures. In the early part of the 21st century, imaging for acute pulmonary embolism improved dramatically, and data emerged suggesting that early surgical intervention for patients with massive or submassive pulmonary emboli resulted in a 93% survival to discharge.[6] From that point, surgeons and researchers began to explore the possibility of surgical pulmonary embolectomy as primary therapy for pulmonary embolism.

INDICATIONS

Historically, surgical pulmonary embolectomy was reserved as a salvage procedure for patients who either failed or had an absolute contraindication to thrombolysis. Given recent advances in surgical technique and technology, surgical pulmonary embolectomy has proven to be a safe and effective approach for patients with a broad range of presentations associated with pulmonary embolism. At selected centers, surgery is being offered as primary therapy for patients with both submassive and massive pulmonary emboli.

Surgical intervention is usually considered at high-volume centers for high-risk submassive and massive pulmonary emboli. Other indications may include the presence of thrombus in transit, concomitant cardiac pathology (a large patent foramen ovale, for instance), or relative contraindications to lytics including recent surgery. In patients who cannot undergo thrombolysis, such as those with recent cerebrovascular or intracranial pathology (eg, cerebrovascular accident, transient ischemic attack, trauma, or recent neurosurgery), active bleeding, or absolute contraindications to anticoagulation, surgical embolectomy may be the preferred approach to management.[7,8] Despite improvements in overall care, surgery for acute pulmonary embolism is utilized infrequently.[9]

The 2019 European Society of Cardiology (ESC) guidelines included surgical pulmonary embolectomy in the management of acute pulmonary embolism. The guidelines listed surgery as a class 2a level C recommendation for management of pulmonary embolectomy to be used only as an alternative to rescue thrombolysis in patients with contraindications to thrombolysis and as an equivalent therapy to percutaneous catheter-directed options in this situation.[10] The same guidelines did acknowledge, however, that there have been favorable results in high-risk and intermediate-risk pulmonary embolectomy patients and even went so far as to acknowledge that retrospective studies reveal no difference in mortality between thrombolysis and embolectomy, with a higher stroke and reintervention risk in patients undergoing thrombolysis.

CURRENT SURGICAL APPROACH

The approach to surgical pulmonary embolectomy has been revised since the initial forays by Trendelenburg to incorporate the now ubiquitous cardiopulmonary bypass circuit. Although variations exist, most surgeries for acute pulmonary emboli involve a median sternotomy, central cannulation, and cardiopulmonary bypass with or without cardioplegic arrest. In select patients with hemodynamic instability, skin preparation and draping take place prior to induction of anesthesia such that if the patient were to experience cardiac arrest, emergent initiation of cardiopulmonary bypass would be facilitated.

Once the chest is entered, the pericardium is opened, and the aorta is fully mobilized. After cannulation, cardiopulmonary bypass is initiated, and the patient remains normothermic. If there is a patent foramen ovale and/or thrombus-in-transit, the superior and inferior vena cavae are cannulated to allow for entry into the right atrium. Routine right atrial exploration is not performed. Given adequate exposure, cardioplegic arrest is usually unnecessary. A pledgeted retraction suture is then placed just cephalad to the pulmonary valve, and the main pulmonary artery is incised in a longitudinal fashion. This incision is extended to the bifurcation of the pulmonary artery, and this usually provides sufficient exposure to retrieve embolic material from both pulmonary arterial trees down to the subsegmental level under direct vision. Pulmonary emboli are then carefully extracted using a combination of manual extraction and suction-assisted extraction. If exposure of the right pulmonary arterial tree remains suboptimal, a longitudinal counterincision is created in the right main pulmonary artery in between the aorta and the superior vena cava. Multiple images are shown that demonstrate the amount and appearance of emboli that can be removed using these strategies (**Figs. 1–3**). Once embolic extraction is complete, the arteriotomies are closed with permanent monofilament suture and cardiopulmonary bypass weaned. The thorax is then closed after decannulation and protamine administration. Careful attention to right ventricular function is paid in the perioperative period. Adjunctive maneuvers to improve right ventricular function include increased systemic blood pressure, inotropy, inhaled vasodilatory agents (including nitric oxide and epoprostenol), intra-aortic balloon counterpulsation, extracorporeal membrane oxygenation, and delayed thoracic closure.

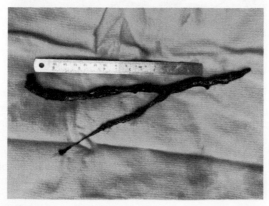

Fig. 1. Pulmonary embolectomy specimen.

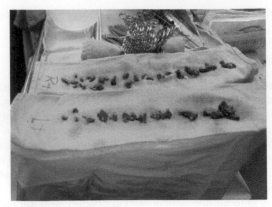

Fig. 2. Specimen after bilateral embolectomy.

SUPPORTING EVIDENCE

The use of surgical pulmonary embolectomy as therapy for acute pulmonary embolism began to reemerge as a valuable treatment modality by 2011, when the American Heart Association released a scientific statement detailing recommendations for appropriate management of pulmonary embolism. In this statement, surgical therapy was highlighted as an effective strategy and recommended this approach in patients with massive pulmonary embolism, submassive pulmonary embolism with right ventricular dysfunction, in patients with right atrial thrombus or paradoxic embolism, and in patients who failed thrombolysis.[11] These recommendations fueled further exploration into the benefits and outcomes of surgical pulmonary embolectomy.

In 2016, Keeling and colleagues[12] published one of the first multicenter experiences with surgical pulmonary embolectomy for acute pulmonary emboli as part of the SPEAR (Surgical Pulmonary Embolectomy as Routine therapy) working group.

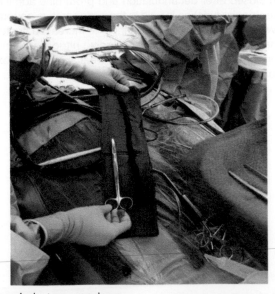

Fig. 3. Pulmonary embolectomy specimen.

Two-hundred and fourteen patients with submassive (82%) or massive (18%) pulmonary emboli were treated with pulmonary embolectomy. This study showed an 11.7% in-hospital mortality, which was significantly lower than previous reports from the iCOPER registry[13] or the Nationwide Inpatient Sample,[14] each of which incompletely evaluated the benefit of surgical therapy for pulmonary embolectomy. This study was also significant in that 28 of the 214 patients (13.1%) had a preoperative cardiac arrest requiring resuscitation, including over one-third of the patients that were diagnosed with massive pulmonary embolism. This speaks to the higher degree of complexity and acuity in the patients who ultimately were considered for surgical pulmonary embolectomy.

In 2017, Kalra and colleagues[15] published a review and comprehensive meta-analysis of 56 studies evaluating the role of surgical pulmonary embolectomy in the treatment of acute pulmonary embolism. They found that the in-hospital all-cause mortality rate of the 1579 patients in all 56 studies was 26.3%, with an in-hospital cardiovascular mortality rate of 14.2% as reported by a combined 45 of 56 studies. Although this was higher than what was reported in the prior multicenter evaluation by Keeling and colleagues, it is worthwhile to note the acuity and severity of the combination of patients in this meta-analysis. Forty-five of 56 studies (involving a total of 1402 patient) reported the incidence of preoperative cardiac arrest, and the combined incidence of preoperative cardiac arrest was 33.9%. Preoperative cardiac arrest is a known risk factor for postoperative mortality following surgical pulmonary embolectomy, and with a third of the cohort experiencing preoperative arrest, it is reasonable to suggest that the overall mortality was significantly affected by this finding.[16] Another important note was that the use of preoperative extracorporeal membrane oxygenation (ECMO) was detailed in 18 of the studies (total of 621 patients), with 27.2% of these patients undergoing initiation of ECMO preoperatively.

Few studies have evaluated longer-term follow-up after surgery for acute pulmonary embolism. Keeling and colleagues[17] performed a single-center retrospective analysis and documented both the short- and midterm echocardiographic data for patients who underwent surgery for acute pulmonary emboli. Notably, there was a single patient who died in the perioperative period (2.3%). Early echo data showed that most patients who underwent surgical embolectomy had immediate and dramatic improvement in right ventricular function, decreased tricuspid regurgitation, and significant lowering of pulmonary arterial pressure (mean pressure 51.2 preoperative, 36.6 postoperative). At a mean follow-up of 30 months, the benefits to right ventricular function persisted. This study highlighted the ability of surgical intervention to provide durable benefit to right ventricular function.

COMPARISONS WITH OTHER THERAPIES

With the re-emergence of surgery as a safe and viable means of treating patients with large pulmonary emboli, multiple studies have compared surgery with other therapies in the treatment of acute pulmonary embolism. One important comparison between surgical embolectomy and thrombolytic therapy was performed by Aymard and colleagues[18] in 2013. This group performed a single-center retrospective analysis of 80 consecutive patients with massive pulmonary embolism who underwent either surgical pulmonary embolectomy or systemic thrombolysis between 2001 and 2007. Of these 80 patients, 28 underwent surgery, and 52 underwent thrombolysis. Early outcomes demonstrated a 3.6% mortality in the surgical cohort, versus a 13.5% mortality in the thrombolysis group. Bleeding complications were noted to be significantly higher in the thrombolysis population (3.6% surgical vs 26.5% thrombolysis).

Neurologic events were likewise higher in the thrombolysis group (20.4%) versus the surgery group (17.9%). At 5-year follow-up, there was no significant mortality difference between the 2 groups, however, with a trend toward better long-term survival in the surgical cohort (17.9% in the surgical group vs 23.1% in the thrombolysis group). This study was one of the first studies directly comparing the 2 treatment modalities and demonstrated that surgical embolectomy can safely be employed as a primary treatment strategy for patients with massive pulmonary emboli.

In 2018, Lee and colleagues[9] performed a retrospective cohort analysis of 2111 patients with acute pulmonary embolism collected from the New York State database between 1999 and 2013. In this study, 88% (n = 1854) received thrombolysis, while only 12% (n = 257) underwent surgical pulmonary embolectomy. The patients who underwent thrombolysis were overall healthier, as fewer had a history of deep vein thrombosis, major surgery, or trauma within 30 days; congestive heart failure; ischemic stroke within 6 months; known coagulopathies; or history of cerebrovascular disease. Patients who underwent thrombolysis were also significantly less likely to have had a previous pulmonary embolism. Despite these differences, there was no difference in 30-day mortality between the groups (thrombolysis 15.2% vs 13.2% for surgery). Thrombolysis was also associated with a significantly higher reintervention rate and stroke rate compared with surgical embolectomy. There was a lower risk of major bleeding with thrombolysis versus surgery. This study also evaluated long-term outcomes and found that there was no difference in the 5-year survival between the groups. Additionally, they found that over 5 years, there was a higher rate of recurrent pulmonary embolism requiring inpatient readmission in the thrombolysis group. There are a few interesting points to highlight from this study. The difference in utilization between the 2 therapies was vast. Also, this study reinforced what has been demonstrated in several studies, that patients who undergo surgery for acute pulmonary embolism have more preoperative comorbidities than patients who undergo other therapeutic interventions. Finally, as Lee and colleagues highlighted, there is more complete clearance of thrombus using a surgical approach, and this may translate to a long-term decrease in recurrent pulmonary emboli and decreased risk for chronic thromboembolic pulmonary hypertension. Overall, this study proved to be encouraging for the future of surgical pulmonary embolectomy, and even initiated early calls for a randomized controlled trial comparing surgical pulmonary embolectomy with thrombolysis and other modalities of therapy to improve overall patient outcomes.[19]

One of the first studies to examine patients who underwent surgery following failed thrombolysis was performed by Meneveau and colleagues[20] in 2006. This group maintained a prospective single-center registry of 488 patients who underwent thrombolytic therapy between 1995 and 2005. Forty of these patients, or 8.2%, did not respond. Unsuccessful thrombolysis within the first 36 hours was defined as both persistent clinical instability (two or more of the following criteria: refractory shock, hypotension, hypoxemia, tachycardia) and residual right ventricular dysfunction on echocardiography. Fourteen of these 40 patients were treated with rescue surgical embolectomy within 72 hours of initial thrombolysis, and 26 patients were treated with repeat thrombolysis at least 24 hours after initial thrombolysis. Patients who underwent salvage surgical embolectomy fared much better than those who underwent repeat thrombolysis. In the embolectomy group, there was 1 death (from refractory cardiogenic shock) and 2 major bleeding episodes in the 14 patients, and 11 of 14 (79%) patients had uneventful postoperative courses. In the repeat thrombolysis group, 10 of 26 (38%) of patients died; 4 patients (15%) had major bleeding episodes (all of which ended in death), and 9 patients (35%) experienced recurrent pulmonary embolism. The patients who died did so because of refractory shock, recurrent embolism, and major bleeding. Only 31% of patients had uneventful postintervention courses. This study highlights that salvage pulmonary embolectomy is an option in patients with failed thrombolysis, and it is likely safer and more efficacious than repeat thrombolysis.

SUMMARY

There is an increasing amount of data to support the use of surgery for patients with large, life-threatening acute pulmonary emboli. As more data continue to support the utilization of surgical intervention for a wide variety of clinical scenarios for patients with acute pulmonary emboli, there is an increasing need for randomized controlled trials comparing surgery with other therapies. As further data accumulate, a greater number of patients will likely derive benefit from surgery after an acute pulmonary embolism.

DISCLOSURE

The authors have nothing to disclose.

REFERENCES

1. Trendelenburg. Über die operative Behandlung der Embolie der Lungenarterie. Arch Klin Chirurg 1908;86:688–700.
2. Sabiston DC Jr. Trendelenburg's classic work on the operative treatment of pulmonary embolism. Ann Thorac Surg 1983;35(5):570–4.
3. Gibbon JH. Artificial maintenance of circulation during experimental occlusion of pulmonary artery. Arch Surg 1937;34:1109.
4. Sharp EH. Pulmonary embolectomy: successful removal of a massive pulmonary embolus with the support of cardiopulmonary bypass: case report. Ann Surg 1962;156:1.
5. Cooley DA, Beall AC, Alexander JK. Acute massive pulmonary embolism. JAMA 1961;177:283–6.
6. Leacche M, Unic D, Goldhaber SZ, et al. Modern surgical treatment of massive pulmonary embolism: results in 47 consecutive patients after rapid diagnosis and aggressive surgical approach. J Thorac Cardiovasc Surg 2005;129: 1018–23.
7. Kon ZN, Pasrija C, Bittle GJ, et al. The incidence and outcomes of surgical pulmonary embolectomy in North America. Ann Thorac Surg 2019;107(5):1401–8.
8. Bloomfield P, Boon NA, de Bono DP. Indications for pulmonary embolectomy. Lancet 1988;2(8606):329.
9. Lee T, Itagaki S, Chiang YP, et al. Survival and recurrence after acute pulmonary embolism treated with pulmonary embolectomy or thrombolysis in New York State, 1999 to 2013. J Thorac Cardiovasc Surg 2018;155(3):1084–90.e12.
10. Konstantinides SV, Meyer G, Beccattini C, et al. 2019 ESC guidelines for the diagnosis and management of acute pulmonary embolism developed in collaboration with the European Respiratory Society (ERS): the task force for the diagnosis and management of acute pulmonary embolism of the European Society of Cardiology (ESC). Eur Heart J 2019;54(3):543–603.
11. Jaff MR, McMurtry MS, Archer SL, et al. Management of massive and submassive pulmonary embolism, iliofemoral deep vein thrombosis, and chronic thromboembolic pulmonary hypertension, a scientific statement from the American Heart Association. Circulation 2011;123:1788–830.

12. Keeling WB, Sundt T, Leacche M, et al. Outcomes after surgical pulmonary embolectomy for acute pulmonary embolus: a multi-institutional study. Ann Thorac Surg 2016;102(5):1498–502.
13. Goldhaber SZ, Visani L, De Rosa M. Acute pulmonary embolism: clinical outcomes in the International Cooperative Pulmonary Embolism Registry (ICOPER). Lancet 1999;353:1386–9.
14. Kilic A, Shah AS, Conte JV, et al. Nationwide outcomes of surgical embolectomy for acute pulmonary embolism. J Thorac Cardiovasc Surg 2013;145:373–7.
15. Kalra R, Bajaj NS, Arora P, et al. Surgical embolectomy for acute pulmonary embolism: systematic review and comprehensive meta-analyses. Ann Thorac Surg 2017;103:982–90.
16. Dauphine C, Omari B. Pulmonary embolectomy for acute massive pulmonary embolism. Ann Thorac Surg 2005;79::1240–4.
17. Keeling WB, Leshnower BG, Lasajanak Y, et al. Midterm benefits of surgical pulmonary embolectomy for acute pulmonary embolus on right ventricular function. J Thorac Cardiovasc Surg 2016;152(3):872–8.
18. Aymard T, Kadner A, Widmer A, et al. Massive pulmonary embolism: surgical embolectomy versus thrombolytic therapy—should surgical indications be revisited? Eur J Cardiothorac Surg 2013;43:90–4.
19. Hirji SA, Kaneko T, Aranki S. Surgical embolectomy for pulmonary embolism: about time for a randomized clinical trial? J Thorac Cardiovasc Surg 2018;155:1080–1.
20. Meneveau N, Séronde MF, Blonde MC, et al. Management of unsuccessful thrombolysis in acute massive pulmonary embolism. Chest 2006;129:1043–50.

Management of Right Ventricular Failure in Pulmonary Embolism

Steven Zhao, MD[a], Oren Friedman, MD[b],*

KEYWORDS

- Pulmonary embolism • Right ventricular failure • Cor pulmonale
- Massive pulmonary embolism • Extracorporeal membrane oxygenation (ECMO)
- Right ventricular support device (RVAD)

KEY POINTS

- Managing hemodynamic compromise from pulmonary embolism (PE) requires knowledge of the pathophysiology of acute right ventricular failure.
- If patients are unstable, prioritize immediate clot reduction via systemic thrombolytics, endovascular procedures, surgical embolectomy, or ECMO.
- Right ventricular failure from PE benefits from addition of systemic vasoconstrictors and inotropes.
- Right ventricular assist devices may have a role in supporting right ventricular failure from PE but more studies are needed.

INTRODUCTION

Significant hemodynamic compromise can be present in as many as 8% of patients with an acute pulmonary embolism (PE). It is associated with a significant increase in mortality from 15% to 42%, which is largely driven by acute right ventricular failure.[1] Management of this complication is predicated on an understanding of the physiology of the right ventricle (RV) in order to carefully support its cardiac output.

PATHOPHYSIOLOGY OF RIGHT VENTRICULAR FAILURE

The RV differs from the left ventricle (LV) in a few key areas. Pulmonary circulatory pressures are markedly lower than those of its systemic counterpart. Accordingly,

[a] Division of Pulmonary and Critical Care medicine, Cedars-Sinai Medical Center, 8700 Beverly Boulevard, Room 6728, Los Angeles, CA 90048, USA; [b] Cedars-Sinai Medical Center, 127 South San Vicente Boulevard, Los Angeles, CA 90048, USA
* Corresponding author.
E-mail address: oren.friedman@cshs.org
Twitter: @orenfriedman (O.F.)

Crit Care Clin 36 (2020) 505–515
https://doi.org/10.1016/j.ccc.2020.02.006
0749-0704/20/© 2020 Elsevier Inc. All rights reserved.

the RV consists of a thin layer of myofibrils arranged in series along the longitudinal axis of the heart, which leads to a chamber that is well suited to accommodate changes in volume but is poorly able to overcome sudden changes in pressure.[2] In patients without preexisting pulmonary vascular disease, the RV is unable to acutely generate pressures of more than 40 mm Hg during systole.[3,4] RV stroke volume decreases precipitously as pulmonary vascular resistance (PVR) increases. First, the RV dilates, and eventually contractility and output decrease. RV dilatation frequently leads to functional tricuspid regurgitation as the tricuspid annulus enlarges. It is crucial to remember that the pulmonary and systemic circulations are inexorably linked. A decrease in RV cardiac output necessitates a decrease in LV cardiac output because the LV cannot pump out any more blood than it receives. In addition, as the dilated RV forces the interventricular septum to bow into the LV it impairs LV filling, a concept known as interventricular dependence. LV filling is therefore reduced both in series (reduced RV output leading to reduced LV filling) and in parallel (through interventricular dependence). Perfusion of the RV occurs during both systole and diastole, and is driven by the gradient between coronary artery pressures and RV transmural pressures.[5] As systemic pressure decreases and RV pressure increases, the RV can become ischemic even in the absence of coronary disease. RV ischemia further worsens RV cardiac output and feeds the cycle. Unless the cycle is broken, there is a risk of progressive hemodynamic collapse.

An acute PE causes a sudden increase in RV afterload, both through direct increases in PVR from clot burden as well as through neurohormonal and hypoxia-mediated feedback mechanisms.[6,7] This process is particularly exemplified by the ability of PEs with low clot burden to still cause a significant increase in RV pressures, and is likely mediated by molecules such as serotonin, thromboxane, and histamine.[8] This increase in PVR leads to an RV pressure and volume overload, which in turn results in a decreased stroke volume. A compensatory neurohormonal cascade increases chronotropy and inotropy, but, because the RV is unable to significantly augment its stroke volume, the primary response to maintain cardiac output is tachycardia. Dilatation of the RV free wall further impairs myocyte function as the chamber moves past the inflection point on its Frank-Starling curve.[5] Meanwhile, leftward displacement of the interventricular septum impairs LV diastolic filling and reduces LV stroke volume.[9] As LV cardiac output decreases, systemic and therefore coronary perfusing pressures decrease too. This reduced coronary perfusing gradient, in combination with inflammatory changes and increased myocardial demand, precipitates RV ischemia. Thus, a feedback loop is generated wherein RV dysfunction begets LV dysfunction, which in turn further injures the RV, forming the so-called RV death spiral[2,10-12] (Fig. 1).

PRELOAD OPTIMIZATION: VOLUME MANAGEMENT

Careful assessment of RV preload is exceedingly important because clinicians must prevent the RV from being preload deficient and also avoid further stress on the failing RV by worsening volume overload. There does not exist a reliable, well-validated standard for predicting volume responsiveness in acute right ventricular failure. Clinical judgment remains paramount, and every patient should be individually assessed.[12] Guidance from studies is limited, as discussed later. This article first explores several common intensive care unit (ICU) measurements used for fluid management in other shock states. Static measurements such as central venous pressure (CVP), although commonly used, have increasingly been shown to be unreliable as a marker of fluid responsiveness, especially in the setting of acutely

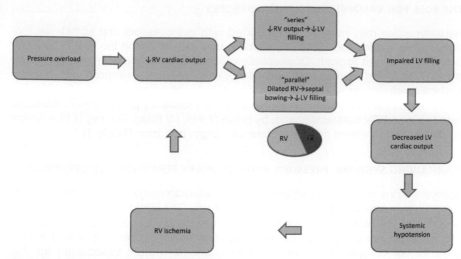

Fig. 1. Physiology of right ventricular failure.

increased right-sided pressures and concomitant increases in tricuspid regurgitation.[13] Furthermore, it is impractical to place a central line for the sole purpose of monitoring CVP in setting of acute PE, as patients will be on anticoagulation and some are being considered for thrombolytics. However, the CVP is a good marker of RV performance. If a patient already has existing central access, an increased CVP usually implies fluid loading will be harmful. Dynamic measurements are generally considered superior to static measurements for predicting fluid responsiveness in shock states; however, many dynamic measurements, such as pulse pressure variation, stroke volume variation, and change in inferior vena cava with positive pressure, are not reliable in the setting of RV dysfunction.[14] Although useful for managing other forms of pulmonary hypertension in the ICU, pulmonary artery (PA) catheters are rarely used in the setting of PE.[15] Data and experience interpreting PA catheter numbers in acute PE are lacking and there is also concern of clot dislodgement and accuracy of pressure measurements in the setting of nonuniform clot distribution in the vascular bed.

A few small nonrandomized studies suggest that, in intermediate-risk PE, treatment with diuresis improved markers of RV strain as well as hemodynamics, whereas other small studies suggest that volume expansion increases cardiac index.[16–18] A prospective multicenter blinded randomized trial is currently ongoing to compare the effects of diuresis and volume expansion in acute intermediate-risk PE.[19] In the interim, the authors favor judicious use of volume expansion to achieve euvolemia, while monitoring for and avoiding other conditions that may excessively reduce RV preload, such as pericardial effusions and cardiac arrhythmias.

EARLY PRIORITY FOR CLOT REDUCTION

Clot debulking treatment via systemic thrombolytics, endovascular procedures, surgery, or otherwise must always be paramount in patients who are hypotensive from PE. Clinicians should evaluate for systemic tissue plasminogen activator long before considering whether to add dobutamine on top of norepinephrine or debating the merits of an inhaled pulmonary vasodilator.

THE ROLE FOR VASOPRESSORS AND INOTROPES

Hemodynamics may need to be supported with vasopressors and sometimes inotropes while waiting for definitive treatment to arrive, or during the time it takes for definitive treatment to work. Occasionally vasoactive medications are needed for residual RV stunning even after clot debulking. Vasopressors are important to maintain systemic perfusion as well as coronary perfusion to the pressure-overloaded RV. The goal is to increase the ratio of systemic vascular resistance (SVR) to PVR. Inotropes help to support RV contractility and, by virtue of this, LV filling. The key is to augment cardiac output to a level commensurate with organ perfusion (**Table 1**).

MAINTAINING SYSTEMIC PRESSURE AND CORONARY PERFUSION: VASOPRESSORS

Norepinephrine is an alpha-adrenergic and beta-adrenergic agent that increases systemic pressure with a modest effect on inotropy. The authors recommend norepinephrine as the first-line agent for shock secondary to PE. Animal studies suggest that norepinephrine improves cardiac output, vascular coupling, and shift tipping point for RV collapse.[20,21] Phenylephrine is another potent vasoconstrictor that has been evaluated for right ventricular failure and can increase RV coronary perfusion, but there is some concern that phenylephrine's pure alpha-adrenergic effect may decrease LV cardiac output.[20,22] Both norepinephrine and phenylephrine have a theoretic possibility of increasing PVR and pressure, but this rarely has practical clinical impact. Norepinephrine has a net benefit favoring an increase in SVR/PVR.[23] One study of patients with chronic pulmonary hypertension undergoing anesthesia suggested a superior hemodynamic response to norepinephrine versus

Table 1 Treatment of acute RV failure		
Goals	**Treatment**	**Comments**
Preload optimization	Judicious volume expansion with crystalloid	• Avoid volume overload • If CVP available and increased, do not give fluids; consider diuretics
Maintain systemic pressure and coronary perfusion	NE 1–40 µg/min is first line	Add vasopressin 0.04 U/min when NE dose >15 µg/min
Augment cardiac output	Dobutamine 2–10 µg/kg/min is first line	• Add dobutamine only after NE has already been started • Avoid milrinone because of vasodilatory effects • Epinephrine 1–10 µg/min is second line
Pulmonary vasodilators	iNO 10–20 ppm or aerosolized epoprostenol 0.03–0.05 µg/kg/min	• Physiologic rationale exists for pulmonary vasodilators • Evidence for benefit is lacking but no indication of harm • Use inhaled pulmonary vasodilators to avoid VQ mismatch

Abbreviations: iNO, inhaled nitric oxide; NE, norepinephrine.

phenylephrine.[24] Vasopressin is a noncatecholamine vasoconstrictor that has a theoretic advantage of increasing SVR without any increase on PVR.[25] The authors recommend its use as a second-line agent when norepinephrine doses exceed 15 μg/min, or if there is a subpar response to norepinephrine. Disadvantages of using vasopressin as a first-line agent include lack of experience, minimal titratability, and absence of inotropic properties.

MAINTAINING CARDIAC OUTPUT: INOTROPES

Inotropes can also improve hemodynamics in the setting of acute unstable PE. The authors suggest the addition of inotropes if there is evidence of a low-cardiac-output state that persists after blood pressure is stabilized with vasopressors. Epinephrine may be useful because it has both vasoconstrictor and inotropic properties.[26] Most clinical experience is with the use of dobutamine. Doses are typically 3 to 5 μg/kg/min, although, rarely, doses up to 10 μg/kg/min are necessary. Dobutamine has been shown to decrease pulmonary arterial elastance and resistance, and to restore RV PA coupling on pressure load–induced right ventricular failure.[27] The authors recommend monitoring metrics of end-organ perfusion such as urine output, mental status, and capillary refill, as well as serial bedside echocardiograms for RV function and cardiac output to help guide titration. Noninvasive cardiac output devices may also be helpful, but many are not accurate in the setting of right ventricular failure. If a central line is in place, measure and target a central venous saturation of 65% to 70% as a resuscitation end point because it reflects oxygen supply and demand. A decrease in central venous saturation reflects cardiac output if hemoglobin level and oxygen consumption are unchanged. Dobutamine does have some vasodilatory properties and can cause hypotension if used alone. However, the hypotensive effects are usually easily balanced out when it is added on top of norepinephrine. In contrast, milrinone is often referred to as an inodilator because of its potent blood pressure lowering effects. Animal models of PE suggest that both dobutamine and milrinone may be effective in improving RV function.[28] Some experts prefer milrinone because of a theoretically reduced risk for tachyarrhythmias and a preferential effect on pulmonary vasodilation.[2,29] However, the potential for hypotension with milrinone is undesirable in the setting of high-risk PE. The authors acknowledge the pulmonary vasodilatory properties of milrinone create a uniquely important role in decompensated pulmonary hypertension but do not recommend its use for acute shock from PE. Levosimendan, a calcium sensitizer that can improve RV inotropy and PVR, is a lesser-known agent that shows some promise in preliminary studies but is currently not approved for use in the United States.[30] Dopamine exerts various effects on cardiac output and vascular tone depending on doses delivered. It has fallen out of favor because of unpredictability, increased arrhythmias, and the availability of superior alternative agents.[31]

When using inotropes, clinicians must monitor closely for arrhythmias because they are both highly prevalent and devastating in patients with acute RV dysfunction.[32] Atrioventricular dissociation is poorly tolerated in acute right ventricular failure. The failing RV becomes dependent on atrial contraction to maintain preload.[33] Sinus tachycardia can increase cardiac output and is beneficial to a point, past which decreased filling time worsens RV and LV preload. Furthermore, excessive tachycardia itself can increase RV myocardial work and further worsen supply-demand mismatch. Digoxin is sometimes used in patients with chronic RV dysfunction from pulmonary hypertension because it increases inotropy without increasing heart rate (and is useful for rate control), but it does not have a role in the acute right ventricular failure setting, and has not been studied in the context of PE.[34]

MANAGING RIGHT VENTRICULAR AFTERLOAD: PULMONARY VASODILATORS

The authors emphasize that the most important method of reducing RV afterload in unstable patients with acute PE involves rapidly reducing clot burden. In stable patients, heparin monotherapy is enough. Heparin alone was shown to reduce PVR by 16% after 24 hours in 1 study.[35] This finding may be caused by heparin's inhibitory effects on platelet aggregation, thus both facilitating clot dissolution and limiting the release of vasoactive substances.[36] In unstable patients, there has been interest in supplementing treatment with pulmonary vasodilators because it is recognized that the increase in PVR following PE is not simply caused by the thrombi themselves but also by the resulting inflammatory and neurohormonal cascade.

Pulmonary vasodilators have long been used to treat pulmonary arterial hypertension. In 1 small randomized study, intravenous (IV) epoprostenol did not significantly improve RV function when combined with usual care for acute PE.[37] Although the use of systemic parenteral therapy has traditionally been limited by concerns of systemic hypotension, inhaled epoprostenol and nitric oxide (iNO) are agents with short half-lives and limited systemic absorption, which makes them attractive targets for use in acute PE.[37,38] Inhaled pulmonary vasodilators are used commonly in unstable patients with various forms of right ventricular failure in combination with increased PVR. In addition to their effects on decreasing PVR, inhaled vasodilators may improve oxygenation through optimization of ventilation/perfusion (V/Q) matching in the lungs. Critically ill patients, including those with acute PE, have V/Q mismatch, so inhaled pulmonary vasodilators are preferred to IV or oral agents. Recently, a randomized, double-blind multicenter study compared administration of inhaled iNO with placebo in patients with intermediate-risk PE.[39] Although the study failed to show a significant difference in the primary outcome (a composite of normal troponin level and RV by echocardiographic criteria), there was a trend toward improvement in echocardiographic parameters of RV dysfunction within 24 hours. There may remain a role for iNO in acute PE, but more robust studies are needed to provide further clarity. For patients who survive the initial PE and subsequently develop chronic thromboembolic pulmonary hypertension, riociguat is an oral pulmonary vasodilator that has been shown to improve hemodynamics and patient symptoms.[40]

MANAGING RESPIRATORY FAILURE: INTUBATION AND MECHANICAL VENTILATION

Patients with PE may develop several indications for intubation and mechanical ventilation. Severe hypoxemia may develop from V/Q mismatch, shunt, and decreased mixed venous oxygen content.[41,42] Contrary to many other groups of critically ill patients, those with acute PE should avoid endotracheal intubation and mechanical ventilation as much as possible because of the high risk of hemodynamic collapse.[43–45] Induction agents used to facilitate intubation may cause a decrease in sympathetic tone and a significant decrease in systemic blood pressures, reducing both RV perfusion and RV preload.[46] In addition, they may also have a direct negative inotropic effect on the myocardium, further decreasing cardiac output. The transient period of apnea may lead to hypoxemia and hypercapnia, both of which may cause an acute increase in PVR.[47,48] Positive pressure ventilation, particularly if tidal volumes are excessively high, may also increase PVR and worsen RV dysfunction.[49] If intubation is deemed necessary, the risk of cardiovascular collapse may be reduced by ensuring close hemodynamic monitoring with vasopressor agents readily available. Potent vasodilators/negative inotropes such as propofol should be avoided, and the most hemodynamically neutral agent, such as etomidate or ketamine, should be considered.[50] One strategy that minimizes the adverse effects of induction agents/sedatives and maximizes the patient's ability to rely on physiologic respiratory mechanics to avoid periprocedural hypotension and hypoxemia is awake fiberoptic intubation. In 1 small case series, patients with acute right heart failure intubated using this strategy had 88% survival in the 24 hours after intubation.[51] When performing fiberoptic intubation in this population, adequate topicalization with lidocaine should be emphasized to reduce abrupt shifts in sympathetic tone from the procedure.[52]

Care should be taken to avoid lung overdistension both while bag masking the patient as well as after the patient is intubated. Notably, both low and high tidal volumes may increase PVR, so avoidance of atelectasis and overdistension is necessary and a lung-protective ventilation strategy similar to that used in acute respiratory distress syndrome (ARDS) may be used.[53] Similarly, higher positive end-expiratory pressure (PEEP) levels may extrinsically compress pulmonary vasculature leading to increases in PVR, whereas its role in alveolar recruitment and improvement of oxygenation may reduce hypoxic vasoconstriction and PVR. No single PEEP strategy has been shown to be preferential in this population, so tidal volumes and PEEP should be carefully titrated for both gas exchange as well as hemodynamics. Prone positioning has been shown to offload the RV in ARDS but that is thought to be related to improved lung recruitment and gas exchange and is not recommended for right ventricular failure from acute PE[54] (**Table 2**).

MANAGING RIGHT VENTRICULAR FAILURE WITH MECHANICAL SUPPORT: EXTRACORPOREAL MEMBRANE OXYGENATION AND RIGHT VENTRICULAR ASSIST DEVICE

In cases of severe shock or hypoxemia refractory to the therapies discussed earlier, mechanical support may be used.[10] This support may be in the form of extracorporeal membrane oxygenation (ECMO) or right ventricular assist device (RVAD). Because circulatory failure predominates over respiratory failure, venoarterial (VA) ECMO is

Table 2
Intubation and mechanical ventilation of patients with acute pulmonary embolism

Goals	Treatment
Avoid intubation if possible	• Treat the underlying cause (PE) first • Respiratory failure should be considered an indication for systemic thrombolytics or other advanced PE treatment • Beware that intubation may precipitate cardiovascular collapse
Cardiostable induction medications	• Use medications with minimal vasodilatory properties • Consider etomidate or ketamine
Maintain systemic blood pressure	• Consider starting norepinephrine before induction • Push-dose phenylephrine is useful
Maintain normoxia and normocarbia	• Hypoxia and hypercapnia lead to an increase in PVR • Attention to preinduction optimization • Minimize apneic period (experienced provider intubates, consider use of video laryngoscopy) • Once intubated, adjust ventilator settings to achieve goals
Optimize tidal volumes	• Tidal volumes too low or too high lead to an increase in PVR • 6–8 mL/kg IBW is a good starting point

Abbreviation: IBW, ideal body weight.

usually considered rather than venovenous ECMO. To date, there have been no prospective studies assessing the role of ECMO in the setting of PE. In a retrospective single-center series, early protocolized use of VA-ECMO resulted in 95% 90-day survival.[55] Patients placed on ECMO were sometimes bridged to definitive therapy with surgical embolectomy or catheter-directed lysis, but many were simply treated with anticoagulation alone. Notably, patients in this series were evaluated for and placed on ECMO early in their course, as opposed to a more traditional use of ECMO as salvage therapy later on. A systematic review of case reports found an overall 70% survival rate, with more than half of those patients receiving ECMO after cardiac arrest.[56] Another less invasive approach may be the use of a percutaneous RVAD.[57,58] One small series examined the use of the Impella RP (a percutaneous microaxial pump that augments RV cardiac output) with catheter-directed thrombolysis with good effect.[59] Akin to ECMO, the goal of a temporary RVADs is to support RV hemodynamics until the acute insult is addressed and PVR is reduced enough to allow weaning and removal. Mechanical support modalities are discussed in greater detail elsewhere in this issue.

SUMMARY

Acute right ventricular failure remains the leading cause of mortality associated with acute PE. Although there is a lack of robust data to guide the management of this critically ill population, clinicians can apply their knowledge of the physiology of the RV and the pathophysiology caused by a PE to tailor therapies toward each patient's needs. First, the clinician must decide on a strategy to debulk clot. The clinician should carefully assess volume status and judiciously resuscitate, being mindful of the harms in volume overloading the RV. Vasopressors are used to increase SVR/PVR, maintain systemic blood pressure, and enhance coronary perfusion to the RV. Inotropes are sometimes needed to maintain adequate cardiac output and LV filling, and improve RV/PA coupling. Pulmonary vasodilators have a theoretic role, but evidence is lacking. Avoid intubation and mechanical ventilation unless it is imperative, applying a physiology-minded approach to both when performed. ECMO has an important role in supporting cardiorespiratory failure from PE, and RVADs may have an expanding role in the future.

DISCLOSURE

Dr O. Friedman is on the speaker's bureau of Bristol Myers Squibb and Pfizer.

REFERENCES

1. Jaff MR, McMurtry MS, Archer SL, et al. Management of massive and submassive pulmonary embolism, iliofemoral deep vein thrombosis, and chronic thromboembolic pulmonary hypertension: a scientific statement from the American Heart Association. Circulation 2011;123(16):1788–830.
2. Ventetuolo CE, Klinger JR. Management of acute right ventricular failure in the intensive care unit. Ann Am Thorac Soc 2014;11(5):811–22.
3. Matthews J, McLaughlin V. Acute right ventricular failure in the setting of acute pulmonary embolism or chronic pulmonary hypertension: a detailed review of the pathophysiology, diagnosis, and management. Curr Cardiol Rev 2008;4(1):49–59.
4. McIntyre KM, Sasahara AA. The hemodynamic response to pulmonary embolism in patients without prior cardiopulmonary disease. Am J Cardiol 1971;28(3): 288–94.

5. Lee FA. Hemodynamics of the right ventricle in normal and disease states. Cardiol Clin 1992;10(1):59–67.
6. Stein M, Levy SE. Reflex and humoral responses to pulmonary embolism. Prog Cardiovasc Dis 1974;17(3):167–74.
7. Malik AB. Pulmonary microembolism. Physiol Rev 1983;63(3):1114–207.
8. Alpert JS, Godtfredsen J, Ockene IS, et al. Pulmonary hypertension secondary to minor pulmonary embolism. Chest 1978;73(6):795–7.
9. Jardin F. Ventricular interdependence: how does it impact on hemodynamic evaluation in clinical practice? Intensive Care Med 2003;29(3):361–3.
10. Konstantinides SV, Torbicki A, Agnelli G, et al. 2014 ESC guidelines on the diagnosis and management of acute pulmonary embolism. Eur Heart J 2014;35(43): 3033–69, 3069a-3069k.
11. Hsu N, Wang T, Friedman O, et al. Medical management of pulmonary embolism: beyond anticoagulation. Tech Vasc Interv Radiol 2017;20(3):152–61.
12. de Asua I, Rosenberg A. On the right side of the heart: medical and mechanical support of the failing right ventricle. J Intensive Care Soc 2017;18(2):113–20.
13. Marik PE, Cavallazzi R. Does the central venous pressure predict fluid responsiveness? An updated metaanalysis and a plea for some common sense. Crit Care Med 2013;41(7):1774.
14. Wyler von Ballmoos M, Takala J, Roeck M, et al. Pulse-pressure variation and hemodynamic response in patients with elevated pulmonary artery pressure: a clinical study. Crit Care 2010;14(3). https://doi.org/10.1186/cc9060.
15. Evans DC, Doraiswamy VA, Prosciak MP, et al. Complications associated with pulmonary artery catheters: a comprehensive clinical review. Scand J Surg 2009;98(4):199–208.
16. Schouver ED, Chiche O, Bouvier P, et al. Diuretics versus volume expansion in acute submassive pulmonary embolism. Arch Cardiovasc Dis 2017;110(11):616–25.
17. Ternacle J, Gallet R, Mekontso-Dessap A, et al. Diuretics in normotensive patients with acute pulmonary embolism and right ventricular dilatation. Circ J 2013; 77(10):2612–8.
18. Mercat A, Diehl JL, Meyer G, et al. Hemodynamic effects of fluid loading in acute massive pulmonary embolism. Crit Care Med 1999;27(3):540–4.
19. Gallet R, Meyer G, Ternacle J, et al. Diuretic versus placebo in normotensive acute pulmonary embolism with right ventricular enlargement and injury: a double-blind randomised placebo controlled study. Protocol of the DiPER study. BMJ Open 2015;5(5):1–6.
20. Hirsch LJ, Rooney MW, Wat SS, et al. Norepinephrine and phenylephrine effects on right ventricular function in experimental canine pulmonary embolism. Chest 1991;100(3):796–801.
21. Molloy WD, Lee KY, Girling L, et al. Treatment of shock in a canine model of pulmonary embolism. Am Rev Respir Dis 1984;130(5):870–4.
22. Layish DT, Tapson VF. Pharmacologic hemodynamic support in massive pulmonary embolism. Chest 1997;111(1):218–24.
23. Rich S, Gubin S, Hart K. The effects of phenylephrine on right ventricular performance in patients with pulmonary hypertension. Chest 1990;98(5):1102–6.
24. Kwak YL, Lee CS, Park YH, et al. The effect of phenylephrine and norepinephrine in patients with chronic pulmonary hypertension. Anaesthesia 2002;57(1):9–14.
25. Gordon AC, Wang N, Walley KR, et al. The cardiopulmonary effects of vasopressin compared with norepinephrine in septic shock. Chest 2012;142(3): 593–605.

26. Boulain T, Lanotte R, Legras A, et al. Efficacy of epinephrine therapy in shock complicating pulmonary embolism. Chest 1993;104(1):300–2.
27. Kerbaul F, Rondelet B, Motte S, et al. Effects of norepinephrine and dobutamine on pressure load-induced right ventricular failure. Crit Care Med 2004;32(4): 1035–40.
28. Tanaka H, Tajimi K, Matsumoto A, et al. Vasodilatory effects of milrinone on pulmonary vasculature in dogs with pulmonary hypertension due to pulmonary embolism: a comparison with those of dopamine and dobutamine. Clin Exp Pharmacol Physiol 1990;17(10):681–90.
29. Jardin F, Genevray B, Brun-Ney D, et al. Dobutamine: a hemodynamic evaluation in pulmonary embolism shock. Crit Care Med 1985;13(12):1009–12.
30. Duygu H, Ozerkan F, Zoghi M, et al. Effect of levosimendan on right ventricular systolic and diastolic functions in patients with ischaemic heart failure. Int J Clin Pract 2008;62(2):228–33.
31. De Backer D, Biston P, Devriendt J, et al. Comparison of dopamine and norepinephrine in the treatment of shock. N Engl J Med 2010;362(9):779–89.
32. Tongers J, Schwerdtfeger B, Klein G, et al. Incidence and clinical relevance of supraventricular tachyarrhythmias in pulmonary hypertension. Am Heart J 2007;153(1):127–32.
33. Goldstein JA, Barzilai B, Rosamond TL, et al. Determinants of hemodynamic compromise with severe right ventricular infarction. Circulation 1990;82(2): 359–68.
34. Rich S, Seidlitz M, Dodin E, et al. The short-term effects of digoxin in patients with right ventricular dysfunction from pulmonary hypertension. Chest 1998;114(3): 787–92.
35. Hirsh J, McDonald IG, Hale GA, et al. Comparison of the effects of streptokinase and heparin on the early rate of resolution of major pulmonary embolism. Can Med Assoc J 1971;104(6):488–91, passim.
36. Mlczoch J, Tucker A, Weir K, et al. Platelet-mediated pulmonary hypertension and hypoxia during pulmonary microembolism. Reduction by platelet inhibition. Chest 1978;74(6):648–53.
37. Kooter AJ, IJzerman RG, Kamp O, et al. No effect of epoprostenol on right ventricular diameter in patients with acute pulmonary embolism: a randomized controlled trial. BMC Pulm Med 2010;10. https://doi.org/10.1186/1471-2466-10-18.
38. Szold O, Khoury W, Biderman P, et al. Inhaled nitric oxide improves pulmonary functions following massive pulmonary embolism: a report of four patients and review of the literature. Lung 2006;184(1):1–5.
39. Kline JA, Puskarich MA, Jones AE, et al. Inhaled nitric oxide to treat intermediate risk pulmonary embolism: a multicenter randomized controlled trial. Nitric Oxide 2019;84:60–8.
40. Ghofrani H-A, D'Armini AM, Grimminger F, et al. Riociguat for the treatment of chronic thromboembolic pulmonary hypertension. N Engl J Med 2013;369(4): 319–29.
41. Huet Y, Lemaire F, Brun-Buisson C, et al. Hypoxemia in acute pulmonary embolism. Chest 1985;88(6):829–36.
42. Santolicandro A, Prediletto R, Fornai E, et al. Mechanisms of hypoxemia and hypocapnia in pulmonary embolism. Am J Respir Crit Care Med 1995;152(1):336–47.
43. McGlothlin D, Ivascu N, Heerdt PM. Anesthesia and pulmonary hypertension. Prog Cardiovasc Dis 2012;55(2):199–217.
44. Friedman O, Horowitz JM, Ramzy D. Advanced cardiopulmonary support for pulmonary embolism. Tech Vasc Interv Radiol 2017;20(3):179–84.

45. Hoeper MM, Granton J. Intensive care unit management of patients with severe pulmonary hypertension and right heart failure. Am J Respir Crit Care Med 2011; 184(10):1114–24.
46. Höhn L, Schweizer A, Morel DR, et al. Circulatory failure after anesthesia induction in a patient with severe primary pulmonary hypertension. Anesthesiology 1999;91(6):1943–5.
47. Lambermont B, Ghuysen A, Janssen N, et al. Comparison of functional residual capacity and static compliance of the respiratory system during a positive end-expiratory pressure (PEEP) ramp procedure in an experimental model of acute respiratory distress syndrome. Crit Care 2008;12(4):R91.
48. Viitanen A, Salmenperä M, Heinonen J. Right ventricular response to hypercarbia after cardiac surgery. Anesthesiology 1990;73(3):393–400.
49. Schulman DS, Biondi JW, Matthay RA, et al. Effect of positive end-expiratory pressure on right ventricular performance. Importance of baseline right ventricular function. Am J Med 1988;84(1):57–67.
50. Stollings JL, Diedrich DA, Oyen LJ, et al. Rapid-sequence intubation: a review of the process and considerations when choosing medications. Ann Pharmacother 2014;48(1):62–76.
51. Johannes J, Berlin DA, Patel P, et al. A technique of awake bronchoscopic endotracheal intubation for respiratory failure in patients with right heart failure and pulmonary hypertension. Crit Care Med 2017;45(9):e980–4.
52. Maxwell BG, Pearl RG, Kudelko KT, et al. Case 7 - 2012 airway management and perioperative decision making in the patient with severe pulmonary hypertension who requires emergency noncardiac surgery. J Cardiothorac Vasc Anesth 2012; 26(5):940–4.
53. Fischer LG, Van Aken H, Bürkle H. Management of pulmonary hypertension: physiological and pharmacological considerations for anesthesiologists. Anesth Analg 2003;96(6):1603–16.
54. Vieillard-Baron A, Charron C, Caille V, et al. Prone positioning unloads the right ventricle in severe ARDS. Chest 2007;132(5):1440–6.
55. Pasrija C, Kronfli A, George P, et al. Utilization of veno-arterial extracorporeal membrane oxygenation for massive pulmonary embolism. Ann Thorac Surg 2018;105(2):498–504.
56. Yusuff HO, Zochios V, Vuylsteke A. Extracorporeal membrane oxygenation in acute massive pulmonary embolism: a systematic review. Perfusion 2015;30(8):611–6.
57. Elder M, Blank N, Shemesh A, et al. Mechanical circulatory support for high-risk pulmonary embolism. Interv Cardiol Clin 2018;7(1):119–28.
58. Anderson MB, Goldstein J, Milano C, et al. Benefits of a novel percutaneous ventricular assist device for right heart failure: the prospective RECOVER RIGHT study of the Impella RP device. J Heart Lung Transplant 2015;34(12):1549–60.
59. Shokr M, Rashed A, Mostafa A, et al. Impella RP support and catheter-directed thrombolysis to treat right ventricular failure caused by pulmonary embolism in 2 patients. Tex Heart Inst J 2018;45(3):182–5.

Supportive Therapy
Extracorporeal Membrane Oxygenation

Vanessa M. Bazan, BSc[a], Peter Rodgers-Fischl, MD[b],
Joseph B. Zwischenberger, MD[c],*

KEYWORDS

- Extracorporeal membrane oxygenation (ECMO) • Pulmonary embolism (PE)
- Hemodynamic instability

KEY POINTS

- The spectrum of pulmonary embolism (PE) ranges from subclinical microemboli to massive embolism causing immediate cardiac arrest.
- Venoarterial extracorporeal membrane oxygenation can be used in the management of high-risk PE with hemodynamic instability as a bridge to treatment or recovery.

INTRODUCTION

After witnessing the sudden death of a patient from acute pulmonary embolism (PE), Dr John Gibbon worked decades to develop cardiopulmonary bypass (CPB).[1] Now, approximately 70 years after his rudimentary CPB circuit first supported open heart surgery, modern versions are used worldwide daily for cardiac surgery and extracorporeal membrane oxygenation (ECMO). ECMO is a modified CPB circuit that

1. Drains venous blood
2. Pumps the blood through a membrane oxygenator where up to full gas exchange occurs
3. Returns the blood to either venous circulation for respiratory support only (venovenous [VV]-ECMO) or arterial circulation for both respiratory and hemodynamic support (venoarterial [VA]-ECMO). Although available for more than 40 years, over the past decade, ECMO has gained popularity for PE resuscitation in the most severe acute PE cases.

Acute PE is a relatively common emergency, with an annual incidence of approximately 1 per 1000 people in the United States.[2,3] Clinical presentation of acute PE

---

[a] College of Medicine, University of Kentucky, Lexington, 800 Rose Street, MN264, Lexington, KY 40536-0298, USA; [b] Division of Cardiothoracic Surgery, Kentucky Clinic, UK Health Care, 740 South Limestone A-301, Lexington, KY 40536, USA; [c] Department of Surgery, University of Kentucky, University of Kentucky Medical Center, 800 Rose Street, MN350, Lexington, KY 40536-0298, USA
* Corresponding author.
E-mail address: joseph.zwischenberger@uky.edu

Crit Care Clin 36 (2020) 517–529
https://doi.org/10.1016/j.ccc.2020.02.007
0749-0704/20/© 2020 Elsevier Inc. All rights reserved.

ranges from absent or mild symptoms (chest pain and cough) to life-threatening hemodynamic deterioration.[4] Acute PE is classified as high risk, intermediate risk, or low risk, based on the degree of hemodynamic compromise.[4] High-risk PE causes hemodynamic instability (shock or hypotension: systolic blood pressure <90 mm Hg or heart rate <40 bpm); intermediate-risk PE causes myocardial strain (identified by echocardiography or elevated plasma troponin or natriuretic peptide levels); and low-risk PE does not cause hemodynamic compromise.

The preferred method of diagnosis for all risk levels of PE is computed tomography (CT) angiography.[4] If CT angiography is unavailable or if a patient is too unstable to be transported to the radiology suite, bedside echocardiography is performed. Low-risk and intermediate-risk PE require anticoagulants, which decrease new thrombus formation and permit existing clot to naturally dissolve.[5] High-risk hemodynamically unstable PE may be treated either with thrombolytics to dissolve clot or embolectomy to remove clot. Current guidelines suggest systemic or catheter-directed thrombolytics as first-line therapy for high-risk PE.[4] Thrombolytics, however, carry a substantial risk of major bleeding and intracerebral hemorrhage and use typically is considered on a case-by-case basis.[6–8] In patients with refractory circulatory collapse or cardiac arrest, ECMO is considered in combination with catheter-directed treatment or surgical embolectomy.[4] Resuscitation or stabilization with VA-ECMO (which provides up to total cardiopulmonary support) prior to surgical embolectomy has improved outcomes over embolectomy alone. See **Table 1** for details. Likewise, several single-center and multicenter reports have demonstrated success with ECMO as a bridge to decision: either surgical embolectomy or as definitive treatment.[9,10] This article reviews the growing literature of ECMO management of PE.

CARDIAC ARREST

Cardiac arrest is an ever-present threat in high risk PE. When emboli obstruct blood flow to the lungs, the increased impedance and resistance elevates right heart pressure, which can rapidly progress to right heart failure with cardiac arrest. The rapidity of deterioration is directly related to the size and amount of obstruction and the degree of stabilization achieved by compensatory physiology. Hemodynamic deterioration to cardiac arrest can occur with large saddle emboli obstructing the bifurcation of the pulmonary artery (**Fig. 1**).[11]

Cardiac arrest during high-risk PE that is refractory to fluids, inotropes, and CPR usually requires immediate CPB or VA-ECMO for salvage.[12,13] ECMO during cardiopulmonary resuscitation (CPR) is known as ECPR and can be initiated in or out of the hospital.[14,15] The goal of ECPR is maintain tissue perfusion during refractory cardiac arrest in order to prevent long-term ischemic damage. Prehospital cardiac arrest has a poor overall survival rate of 6% to 15%[16–18] whereas in-hospital cardiac arrest from PE has a survival rate of 25% when supported with ECPR.[19] As in all major series, improved survival is related directly to timely initiation of resuscitation and ECMO.

As discussed previously, the most important determinant of ECPR outcome is early initiation of quality chest compressions to generate a modest cardiac output (low-flow) that supplies coronary blood flow, facilitating the return of spontaneous circulation (ROSC).[20–22] ECPR should be considered only when CPR is initiated within 5 minutes of cardiac arrest.[15] A 6-year (2005–2011) retrospective registry study capturing all prehospital cardiac arrests in Denmark (Danish Cardiac Arrest Registry) demonstrated bystander CPR initiated within 5 minutes of arrest doubled 30-day survival from 6.3% (no bystander CPR; 95% CI, 5.1–7.6) to 14.5% (95% CI, 12.8–16.4).[20,23]

Table 1
Recent reports of extracorporeal membrane oxygenation for pulmonary embolism

Author	Date	Extracorporeal Membrane Oxygenation (n)	Indications for Extracorporeal Membrane Oxygenation	Pre–extracorporeal Membrane Oxygenation Cardiac Arrest (n)	Pre–extracorporeal Membrane Oxygenation Treatment (n)	Survival, % (n)	Definitive Therapy, n (Discharged [n])
Al-Bawardy et al,[42] 2019	2012–2019	13	RV dilatation and RV hypokinesis	13	NR	69 (7/13), 30-d overall	1 anticoagulation (1, 90-d) 8 systemic thrombolytics (3, 90-d) 3 catheter-directed thrombolytics (1, 90-d) 4 surgical embolectomy (2, 90-d)
Ius et al,[26] 2019	2012–2018	36	Cardiac arrest or refractory hemodynamic instability	15	19 thrombolytics or catheter-directed therapy	67 (24/36) to discharge	16 anticoagulation (5) 9 failed on ECMO 7 decannulated 20 surgical embolectomy (19)

(continued on next page)

Table 1
(continued)

Author	Date	Extracorporeal Membrane Oxygenation (n)	Indications for Extracorporeal Membrane Oxygenation	Pre–extracorporeal Membrane Oxygenation Cardiac Arrest (n)	Pre–extracorporeal Membrane Oxygenation Treatment (n)	Survival, % (n)	Definitive Therapy, n (Discharged [n])
Kjaergaard et al,[43] 2019	2004–2017	22	Cardiac arrest	22	5 thrombolytics	92 (13/14) never ECMO, 30-d 54 (12/22) ECMO, 30-d	10 anticoagulation (4, 30-d) 1 failed on ECMO from incorrect cannulation 7 thrombolytics (2, 30-d) 5 surgical embolectomy (3, 30-d) 14 thrombolytics, never ECMO (13, 30-d)
Kmiec etal,[41] 2020	2006–2017	75 VA-ECMO 46 VV-ECMO 29	VA: cardiac arrest, RV failure with refractory hemodynamic instability VV: respiratory failure refractory to mechanical ventilation	49	23 thrombolytics	47 (35/75) to discharge	28 anticoagulation 7 thrombolytics 8 interventional thrombectomy 10 surgical embolectomy

Study	Type	Years	N	Indication		Treatment	Survival %	Details
Pasrija et al,[9] 2018	Protocol	2015–2017	27	Massive PE with unknown neurologic status or end-organ dysfunction	6	6 thrombolytics	97 (28/29) to discharge	15 anticoagulation (14), 1 confirmed neurologic death, 12 surgical embolectomy (12), 2 surgical embolectomy, never ECMO
	Historic	2011–2015	6	Cardiac arrest before planned surgical embolectomy	6	NR	82 (22/27) to discharge	6 surgical embolectomy, 27 surgical embolectomy, never ECMO
Pasrija et al,[10] 2018		2014–2016	20	Massive PE with unknown neurologic status or end-organ dysfunction	5	7 thrombolytics	95 (19/20) to discharge	8 anticoagulation (7), 1 confirmed neurologic death, 11 surgical embolectomy (11), 1 catheter-directed thrombolytics (1)
George et al,[19] 2018		2012–2015	32	Massive PE with hemodynamic instability or end-organ dysfunction	15	NR	53 (17/32) to discharge	5 systemic thrombolysis (0), 15 catheter-directed thrombolytics (11), 4 aspiration thrombectomy (3), 2 surgical embolectomy (0)

(continued on next page)

Table 1
(continued)

Author	Date	Extracorporeal Membrane Oxygenation (n)	Indications for Extracorporeal Membrane Oxygenation	Pre–extracorporeal Membrane Oxygenation Cardiac Arrest (n)	Pre–extracorporeal Membrane Oxygenation Treatment (n)	Survival, % (n)	Definitive Therapy, n (Discharged [n])
Meneveau et al,[29] 2018	2014–2015	52	Cardiac arrest, hemodynamic instability, contraindication to of failure of other therapies, failure to wean CPB	39	17 thrombolytics 10 surgical embolectomy	38, 30-d	18 anticoagulation (4) 7 surgical embolectomy (4)
Corsi et al,[11] 2017	2006–2015	17	Cardiac arrest, cardiogenic shock	15	8 thrombolytics 2 surgical embolectomy 1 catheter-directed thromboaspiration	47 (8/17) to discharge	6 anticoagulation 1 catheter-directed thromboaspiration 1 surgical embolectomy
Swol et al,[44] 2016	2008–2014	5	Cardiac arrest	5	All surgical patients	40 (2/5) to discharge	3 systemic thrombolytics (1) 1 surgical embolectomy (0)

Abbreviation: NR, not reported.

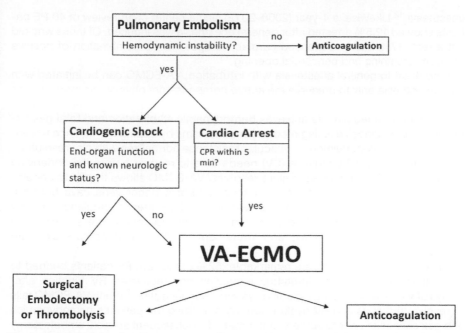

Fig. 1. Hemodynamic deterioration to cardiac arrest can occur with large saddle emboli obstructing the bifurcation of the pulmonary artery. (*Data from* Corsi F, Lebreton G, Bréchot N, et al. Life-threatening massive pulmonary embolism rescued by venoarterial-extracorporeal membrane oxygenation. Crit Care. 2017;21:76.)

When time between arrest and CPR increased to 10 minutes, 30-day survival dropped to 6.7% (95% CI, 5.4–8.1) but showed a 3-fold survival benefit compared with no bystander CPR. After 13 minutes, the association between survival and bystander CPR was no longer significant.[20]

If CPR fails to achieve ROSC after 10 minutes of refractory arrest in qualified patients, tissue reperfusion with ECPR cannulation should occur with VA-ECMO.[15,24] Reynolds and colleagues[21] showed if ROSC is not achieved within 16 minutes of CPR, survival with good neurologic outcome drops below 2%. Likewise, Sakuma and colleagues[25] reported ECPR survival less than 10% when CPR duration was longer than 30 minutes. These data support the concept that just a few minutes either way are critical to quality survival.

CARDIOGENIC SHOCK

Survival drops below 10% when ECMO is initiated 30-minutes postarrest,[25] yet survival as high as 76% has been reported when ECMO is started before cardiac arrest during progressive cardiogenic shock.[19] Attempts to stabilize rapid deterioration during PE-induced cardiogenic shock can counterintuitively compound deterioration. During a PE, induction of general anesthesia with endotracheal intubation counteracts the body's vasoactive compensatory mechanisms, causing vasodilation and decreased mean blood pressure. Additionally, positive pressure ventilation decreases venous return and further accelerates hypotension with risk of sudden cardiac arrest.[12,26] A 10-year single-center chart review of 57 consecutive PE patients reported 19% experienced immediate hypotension and cardiac arrest after induction of general anesthesia.[12] Likewise, a 4-year (2008–2012) single-center chart review of 40 PE patients showed 12.5% arrested after general anesthesia was induced. Of those who did not arrest, 17% later experienced cardiac collapse from a combination of positive pressure breathing and pericardial opening.[13]

In contrast to general anesthesia with intubation, VA-ECMO can be initiated with local anesthesia only to preserve the active compensatory physiologic mechanisms and avoid an unpredictable cardiac arrest. VA-ECMO with systemic anticoagulation and heparin-bonded circuits achieves hemodynamic stabilization and total gas exchange and enhances existing recovery mechanisms by tipping the balance toward thrombus resolution. Pulmonary vascular resistance normalizes with clot resolution, but the distended right ventricle (RV) needs time to recover before the underlying threat of arrest from right heart failure resolves. VA-ECMO allows the RV to decompress by removing volume from the inferior and/or superior vena cava before it reaches the right heart. Blood then is returned to the systemic circulation, usually by femoral artery access. If the right heart does not decompress, additional venous drainage, higher flow, and trans-septal left atrial decompression are options.[27]

The benefits of VA-ECMO are remarkable; 52% of massive PE patients bridged to surgical embolectomy had thrombus resolution and recovered RV function after 3 days of VA-ECMO support, including systemic heparinization.[9] When VA-ECMO fails to resolve thrombus and RV dysfunction, by stabilizing the patient's hemodynamics and gas exchange prior to surgery, outcomes of a subsequent surgical embolectomy may improve. Pasrija and colleagues[10] showed massive PE supported with VA-ECMO (n = 20) before surgical embolectomy had 95% in-hospital survival (100% survival after decannulation), with 40% of patients recovering with VA-ECMO support alone. Systemic thrombolytics typically are not given concomitantly with VA-ECMO; however, catheter-directed thrombolysis while on VA-ECMO has been reported.[19] ECMO also has been used successfully for stabilization before catheter-directed thrombolysis.[28]

Table 1 summarizes the current literature regarding ECMO support for acute PE. Studies include case series and cohort studies, ranging from 5 patients to 75 patients. There currently are no randomized control trials comparing VA-ECMO to medical therapy or surgical embolectomy alone for acute PE. The table illustrates the complex decision making and lack of consensus regarding patient selection and timing of VA-ECMO. The most common indication for VA-ECMO in acute PE was cardiac arrest with study groups containing 25% to 100% of pre-ECMO cardiac arrest. Once ECMO was initiated, patients were bridged to anticoagulation, systemic thrombolytics, catheter-directed thrombolytics, and surgical embolectomy, alone or in combination. Survival ranged from 38% to 97%.[9,29]

PREGNANCY

PE is a leading cause of death during pregnancy.[30] ECMO should be considered for massive PE during pregnancy because the stability of the mother and the survival of the child depend on adequate perfusion and gas exchange. Maternal blood gases of Pao_2 greater than or equal to 70 mm Hg, oxygen saturation greater than or equal to 95%, and $Paco_2$ 30 mm Hg to 32 mm Hg[31] are proposed to ensure survival of both child and mother. Through decades of experience with CPB during pregnancy, and multiple cases of ECMO, the use of heparin anticoagulation during pregnancy has been established as relatively safe.[32–35] Low-molecular-weight heparin and unfractionated heparin do not cross the placenta and are the drugs of choice for PE during pregnancy.[35] In contrast, thrombolytics are relatively contraindicated in pregnancy and are associated with higher postpartum hemorrhage.[36]

CANNULATION STRATEGIES

VA-ECMO is the most common ECMO strategy for supporting massive PE. For patients with hemodynamic instability, cannulation for VA-ECMO often is performed emergently. The most commonly employed cannulation strategy utilizes femoral venous drainage and femoral arterial return. This strategy is popular because it can be accomplished at the bedside either by a percutaneous approach or with a surgical cutdown for insertion. To prevent vascular complications in the groin when attempting to establish urgent access, preplacement of suture-mediated closure devices (ie, Perclose ProGlide, Abbott Vascular, Santa Clara, CA) has been reported.[37] After femoral arterial access is obtained, an additional distal perfusion cannula (5–6 French) should be routinely placed to prevent distal limb ischemia.[38,39] The importance of distal perfusion is elevated in patients with a history of peripheral vascular disease due to their increased likelihood of vascular complications.[40]

Recently, VV-ECMO has also been used to support PE patients with RV strain secondary to respiratory failure.[41] VV-ECMO requires only venous access to oxygenate and ventilate central venous blood through the ECMO circuit. Although lacking in cardiac support, total gas exchange often stabilizes the patient by relieving pulmonary vasoconstriction and also provides therapeutic systemic anticoagulation, without the increased risk of arterial access. If VV-ECMO fails to

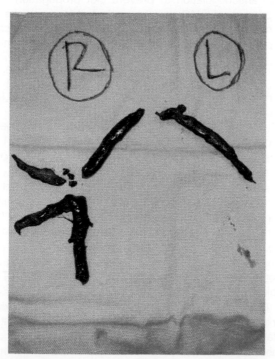

Fig. 2. Saddle embolus surgically removed from right and left pulmonary vessels.

relieve right heart strain and reverse the respiratory failure, conversion to VA-ECMO is accomplished by additional arterial access previously described to achieve cardiac support.

PULMONARY EMBOLISM RESPONSE TEAM

PE response teams (PERTs) are interdisciplinary teams developed to optimize care for PE. The teams may consist of pulmonologists, cardiologists, radiologists, cardiothoracic surgeons, and critical care and emergency medicine physicians.[26,42] Decisions to use advanced treatments are made by the PERT in collaboration with the primary treatment team and the patient's family.[42] The risk-benefit analysis for treatment with thrombolysis, surgical embolectomy, and ECMO is complex and made on a case-by-case basis. The authors have placed the literature experience in a table to illustrate the wide variability of practices, preferences, techniques, and outcomes (see **Table 1**). From this table, it can readily be appreciated that patient selection, use of thrombectomy or anticoagulation prior to ECMO, use of thrombectomy or catheter-based thrombolytics, and patient outcomes are extremely variable, yet promising, toward improved care of saddle embolus. A review of these articles shows the benefit of an algorithm-based management approach of PE (**Fig. 2**). Additional studies are required to define the best algorithms to utilize during different patient presentations.

SUMMARY

Massive PE represents a minority of PE cases but is associated with high mortality. ECMO can stabilize cardiac output and allows gas exchange while simultaneously providing systemic anticoagulation to prevent clot propagation and allow natural thrombolytics to progress. ECMO can be implanted in an awake patient, thereby avoiding hemodynamic collapse from anesthesia. ECMO is indicated as either a bridge to recovery or a decision to perform thrombectomy or thrombolysis.

REFERENCES

1. Hill JD. John H. Gibbon, Jr. Part I. The development of the first successful heart-lung machine. Ann Thorac Surg 1982;34:337–41.
2. Beckman MG, Hooper WC, Critchley SE, et al. Venous thromboembolism: a public health concern. Am J Prev Med 2010;38(4 Suppl):S495–501.
3. Konstantinides SV, Barco S, Lankeit M, et al. Management of pulmonary embolism: an update. J Am Coll Cardiol 2016;67:976–90.
4. Konstantinides SV, Meyer G, Becattini C, et al. 2019 ESC Guidelines for the diagnosis and management of acute pulmonary embolism developed in collaboration with the European Respiratory Society (ERS): the Task Force for the diagnosis and management of acute pulmonary embolism of the European Society of Cardiology (ESC). Eur Heart J 2019;54 [pii:1901647].
5. Furlan A, Aghayev A, Chang CC, et al. Short-term mortality in acute pulmonary embolism: clot burden and signs of right heart dysfunction at CT pulmonary angiography. Radiology 2012;265:283–93.
6. Chatterjee S, Chakraborty A, Weinberg I, et al. Thrombolysis for pulmonary embolism and risk of all-cause mortality, major bleeding, and intracranial hemorrhage: a meta-analysis. JAMA 2014;311:2414–21.
7. Piazza G, Hohlfelder B, Jaff MR, et al. A prospective, single-arm, multicenter trial of ultrasound-facilitated, catheter-directed, low-dose fibrinolysis for acute

massive and submassive pulmonary embolism: the SEATTLE II study. JACC Cardiovasc Interv 2015;8:1382–92.

8. Kucher N, Boekstegers P, Müller OJ, et al. Randomized, controlled trial of ultrasound-assisted catheter-directed thrombolysis for acute intermediate-risk pulmonary embolism. Circulation 2014;129:479–86.

9. Pasrija C, Shah A, George P, et al. Triage and optimization: a new paradigm in the treatment of massive pulmonary embolism. J Thorac Cardiovasc Surg 2018;156: 672–81.

10. Pasrija C, Kronfli A, George P, et al. Utilization of veno-arterial extracorporeal membrane oxygenation for massive pulmonary embolism. Ann Thorac Surg 2018;105:498–504.

11. Corsi F, Lebreton G, Bréchot N, et al. Life-threatening massive pulmonary embolism rescued by venoarterial-extracorporeal membrane oxygenation. Crit Care 2017;21:76.

12. Rosenberger P, Shernan SK, Shekar PS, et al. Acute hemodynamic collapse after induction of general anesthesia for emergent pulmonary embolectomy. Anesth Analg 2006;102:1311–5.

13. Bennett JM, Pretorius M, Ahmad RM, et al. Hemodynamic instability in patients undergoing pulmonary embolectomy: institutional experience. J Clin Anesth 2015;27:207–13.

14. Bělohlávek J, Dytrych V, Linhart A. Pulmonary embolism, part I: epidemiology, risk factors and risk stratification, pathophysiology, clinical presentation, diagnosis and nonthrombotic pulmonary embolism. Exp Clin Cardiol 2013;18:129–38.

15. Hutin A, Abu-Habsa M, Burns B, et al. Early ECPR for out-of-hospital cardiac arrest: best practice in 2018. Resuscitation 2018;130:44–8.

16. Ebner M, Kresoja KP, Keller K, et al. Temporal trends in management and outcome of pulmonary embolism: a single-centre experience. Clin Res Cardiol 2019;109(1):67–77.

17. Bougouin W, Marijon E, Planquette B, et al. Pulmonary embolism related sudden cardiac arrest admitted alive at hospital: management and outcomes. Resuscitation 2017;115:135–40.

18. Pokorna M, Necas E, Skripsky R, et al. How accurately can the aetiology of cardiac arrest be established in an out-of-hospital setting? Analysis by "concordance in diagnosis crosscheck tables. Resuscitation 2011;82:391–7.

19. George B, Parazino M, Omar HR, et al. A retrospective comparison of survivors and non-survivors of massive pulmonary embolism receiving veno-arterial extracorporeal membrane oxygenation support. Resuscitation 2018;122:1–5.

20. Rajan S, Wissenberg M, Folke F, et al. Association of bystander cardiopulmonary resuscitation and survival according to ambulance response times after out-of-hospital cardiac arrest. Circulation 2016;134:2095–104.

21. Reynolds JC, Frisch A, Rittenberger JC, et al. Duration of resuscitation efforts and functional outcome after out-of-hospital cardiac arrest: when should we change to novel therapies? Circulation 2013;128(23):2488–94.

22. Singer B, Reynolds JC, Lockey DJ, et al. Pre-hospital extra-corporeal cardiopulmonary resuscitation. Scand J Trauma Resusc Emerg Med 2018;26:21.

23. Wissenberg M, Lippert FK, Folke F, et al. Association of national initiatives to improve cardiac arrest management with rates of bystander intervention and patient survival after out-of-hospital cardiac arrest. JAMA 2013;310: 1377–84.

24. Kim TH, Shin SD, Kim YJ, et al. The scene time interval and basic life support termination of resuscitation rule in adult out-of-hospital cardiac arrest. J Korean Med Sci 2015;30:104–9.

25. Sakuma M, Nakamura M, Yamada N, et al. Percutaneous cardiopulmonary support for the treatment of acute pulmonary embolism: summarized review of the literature in Japan including our own experience. Ann Vasc Dis 2009;2:7–16.

26. Ius F, Hoeper MM, Fegbeutel C, et al. Extracorporeal membrane oxygenation and surgical embolectomy for high-risk pulmonary embolism. Eur Respir J 2019;53: 1801773.

27. Kapur NK, Paruchuri V, Jagannathan A, et al. Mechanical circulatory support for right ventricular failure. JACC Heart Fail 2013;1:127–34.

28. Weinberg A, Tapson VF, Ramzy D. Massive pulmonary embolism: extracorporeal membrane oxygenation and surgical pulmonary embolectomy. Semin Respir Crit Care Med 2017;38(1):66–72.

29. Meneveau N, Guillon B, Planquette B, et al. Outcomes after extracorporeal membrane oxygenation for the treatment of high-risk pulmonary embolism: a multicentre series of 52 cases. Eur Heart J 2018;39:4196–204.

30. Petersen EE, Davis NL, Goodman D, et al. Vital signs: pregnancy-related deaths, United States, 2011-2015, and strategies for prevention, 13 States, 2013-2017. MMWR Morb Mortal Wkly Rep 2019;68(18):423–9.

31. Whitty JE, Dombrowski MP. Respiratory diseases in pregnancy. In: Resnik R, Lockwood CJ, Moore T, et al, editors. Creasy and Resnik's maternal-fetal medicine: principles and practice. Philidelphia: Elsevier; 2019. p. 1043–66.

32. Taenaka H, Ootaki C, Matsuda C, et al. Successful pulmonary embolectomy for massive pulmonary embolism during pregnancy: a case report. JA Clin Rep 2017;3:44.

33. Brodie D. ECMO in pregnancy and the peripartum period. Qatar Med J 2017; 2017.43.

34. Sharma NS, Wille KM, Bellot SC, et al. Modern use of extracorporeal life support in pregnancy and postpartum. ASAIO J 2015;61:110–4.

35. American College of Obstetricians and Gynecologists. Thromboembolism in pregnancy. ACOG practice bulletin No. 196. American College of Obstetricians and Gynecologists. Obstet Gynecol 2018;132:e1–17.

36. Martillotti G, Boehlen F, Robert-Ebadi H, et al. Treatment options for severe pulmonary embolism during pregnancy and the postpartum period: a systematic review. J Thromb Haemost 2017;15:1942–50.

37. Sakakura K, Adachi Y, Taniguchi Y, et al. Rapid switch from intra-aortic balloon pumping to percutaneous cardiopulmonary support using perclose ProGlide. Case Rep Cardiol 2015;2015:407059.

38. Stulak JM, Dearani JA, Burkhard HM, et al. ECMO cannulation controversies and complications. Semin Cardiothorac Vasc Anesth 2009;12:176–82.

39. Ranney DN, Benrashid E, Meza JM, et al. Vascular complications and use of a distal perfusion cannula in femorally cannulated patients on extracorporeal membrane oxygenation. ASAIO J 2018;64:328–33.

40. Bidas T, Beutel G, Warnecke G, et al. Vascular complications in patients undergoing femoral cannulation for extracorporeal membrane oxygenation support. Ann Thorac Surg 2011;92626–31.

41. Kmiec L, Philipp A, Floerchinger B, et al. Extracorporeal membrane oxygenation for massive pulmonary embolism as bridge to therapy. ASAIO J 2020;66(2): 146–52.

42. Al-Bawardy R, Rosenfield K, Borges J, et al. Extracorporeal membrane oxygenation in acute massive pulmonary embolism: a case series and review of the literature. Perfusion 2019;34:22.
43. Kjaergaard B, Kristensen JH, Sindby JE, et al. Extracorporeal membrane oxygenation in life-threatening massive pulmonary embolism. Perfusion 2019;34:467–74.
44. Swol J, Buchwald D, Strauch J, et al. Extracorporeal life support (ECLS) for cardiopulmonary resuscitation (CPR) with pulmonary embolism in surgical patients - a case series. Perfusion 2016;31:54–9.

Special Considerations in Pulmonary Embolism

Clot-in-Transit and Incidental Pulmonary Embolism

Christopher Kabrhel, MD, MPH[a],*, Rachel Rosovsky, MD, MPH[b],
Shannon Garvey, MS[c]

KEYWORDS

- Pulmonary embolism • Clot-in-transit • Venous thromboembolism

KEY POINTS

- Clot-in-transit (CIT) describes a venous thromboembolism that has become lodged in the right heart.
- CIT is associated with high mortality and presents unique challenges in management.
- Incidental pulmonary embolism (IPE) describes PE diagnosed on imaging performed for another (non-PE) indication.
- The treatment of these patients is complex because there is often a disconnect between the severity of the PE on imaging and the (lack of) severity of the clinical presentation.

INTRODUCTION

This article focuses on 2 relatively rare, but complex situations faced by clinicians treating patients with pulmonary embolism (PE): clot-in-transit (CIT), incidental PE (IPE). CIT describes a venous thromboembolism (VTE) that has become lodged in the right heart. CIT is associated with high mortality and presents unique challenges in management. IPE describes PE diagnosed on imaging performed for another (non-PE) indication. The treatment of these patients is complex because there is often a disconnect between the severity of the PE on imaging and the (lack of) severity of the clinical presentation. Unfortunately, there are not robust data that define the optimal approach to either of these situations. However, in the discussion that follows, our

[a] Department of Emergency Medicine, Center for Vascular Emergencies, Massachusetts General Hospital, Harvard Medical School, Zero Emerson Place, Suite 3B, Boston, MA 02114, USA; [b] Division of Hematology, Department of Medicine, Massachusetts General Hospital, 55 Fruit Street, Boston, MA 02114, USA; [c] Boston University School of Medicine, 72 E Concord Street, Boston, MA 02118, USA
* Corresponding author.
E-mail address: ckabrhel@mgh.harvard.edu

Crit Care Clin 36 (2020) 531–546
https://doi.org/10.1016/j.ccc.2020.02.008
0749-0704/20/© 2020 Elsevier Inc. All rights reserved.

criticalcare.theclinics.com

goal was to summarize the available literature and aid clinicians as they manage patients with PE across the clinical severity spectrum.

CLOT-IN-TRANSIT

CIT is a rare but clinically important manifestation of VTE with increased mortality compared with PE alone.[1] In CIT, a thromboembolus from the deep veins is temporarily lodged in the right heart before entering the pulmonary vasculature. CIT, when left untreated, is associated with mortality rates between 80% and 100%, with one study reporting 100% of deaths in patients with CIT occurring within 24 hours of diagnosis.[2–5] Therefore, it is important that we understand the risk factors and pathophysiology of CIT so we can make rapid diagnoses and initiate appropriate treatment.

EPIDEMIOLOGY

In published studies, the prevalence of CIT ranges from 3% among all patients with acute PE.[6] However, the prevalence of CIT is higher among patients with a more severe PE population, and may occur in as many as 18% of patients with "massive," hemodynamically unstable, PE.[7] In recent years, the incidence of CIT appears to be increasing, possibly due to the increased use of cardiac echocardiography for the prognostic assessment of confirmed PE and improvements in imaging technology.[8] Age and sex do not seem to be associated with CIT.[6,9,10]

TYPES OF RIGHT HEART THROMBI

The European Working Group on Echocardiography has classified 3 types of right heart thrombi. *Type A* thrombi are known as CITs.[11] They are thought to have embolized from the deep veins, traveled through the venous circulation, and become temporarily lodged in the right heart before entering the pulmonary vasculature. A CIT can be located in the right atrium or right ventricle and may prolapse across the tricuspid valve or pulmonic valve during the cardiac cycle.[5] Thrombi visualized in the superior or inferior vena cava also qualify as CITs.[12] A subtype of CIT is a thrombus that has become fixed in a patent foramen ovale or septal defect. These CITs extend into the left side of the heart and can lead to paradoxic embolism. Morphologically, CITs are described as highly mobile, serpiginous masses that are free-floating or have a thin point of attachment (**Fig. 1**A, B) and refer to the CT scan images.[5,11] If a CIT becomes attached to intracardiac structures, such as the Eustachian valve, tricuspid apparatus, or ventricular trabeculae, it may have a pedunculated morphology.[13] CITs are highly associated with PE and are associated with high mortality; however, they are not associated with other thrombogenic cardiac abnormalities or dysrhythmias.[11]

Type B thrombi are known as mural thrombi. Mural thrombi demonstrate similar characteristics to left heart thrombi.[11] They are immobile with a broad-based attachment to the right atrial or right ventricular wall and are thought to have formed in situ.[5] Mural thrombi are associated with thrombogenic cardiac abnormalities, such as atrial fibrillation, right atrial enlargement, foreign bodies in the right heart (pacemaker wire, central venous line, and ventriculo-atrial shunts), atriotomy, and right ventricular damage (infarction, congestive cardiomyopathy, and chronic right heart failure).[11] They have a relatively low mortality rate and are less likely to be associated with PE.[11]

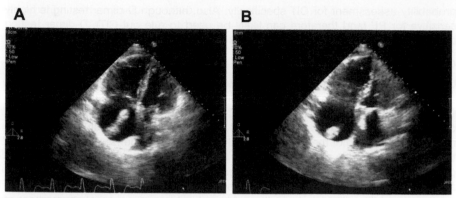

Fig. 1. (*A, B*) Mobile CIT in the right atrium.

Type C thrombi exhibit intermediate characteristics and are described as resembling myxomas.[11]

PATHOPHYSIOLOGY

Because CIT is a manifestation of VTE, the main risk factors and pathogenesis of CIT are similar to those of VTE. The elements of the Virchow Triad that contribute to the development of VTE include multiple genetic and environmental risk factors that promote thrombogenesis.[14] Oftentimes, patients with VTE possess multiple risk factors.[15] Similar to VTE, recent studies have found immobilization to be a common risk factor among patients with CIT.[2,6] In addition, CIT has been associated with a number of hypercoagulable states, including antiphospholipid antibody syndrome, protein C and protein S deficiency, antithrombin III deficiency, and Bechet disease.[2,16]

Few risk factors differentiating CIT from VTE without CIT have been described. Studies have found CIT to be more common among patients with congestive heart failure (CHF).[6,10,17] It is thought that CHF promotes stasis within a dilated and hypokinetic right heart entrapping the VTE or encouraging in situ thrombosis instigated by the thrombogenesis of the VTE event.[1,10] Studies have also found CIT to be more common among patients with severe PE.[7,9,10] It is thought that the elevated pulmonary artery pressures associated with more severe PE create a right to left gradient that halts the VTE as it passes through the heart and prevents it from migrating into the pulmonary vasculature.[10,18]

Clinical Presentation

Dyspnea is the most common presenting symptom in patients with CIT, followed by chest pain and syncope/presyncope.[2–7,10,13,17,19–21] These symptoms present in CIT with frequencies similar to PE without CIT, although one study by Torbicki and colleagues[6,10,21] found that these symptoms progress more quickly in patients with CIT. Similarly, patients with CIT are more likely to present with signs of more severe PE: right ventricular dysfunction and hemodynamic instability.[6,9,10,21]

DIAGNOSIS

In the diagnosis of PE, the first step is the assessment of pretest probability, followed by a combination of D-dimer testing and computed tomography pulmonary angiography (CTPA). Unfortunately, there are no clinical assessment tools to guide pretest probability assessment for CIT specifically. Also, although D-dimer testing is highly sensitive for PE (and therefore can likely be used to rule out CIT), D-dimer testing cannot distinguish between patients with acute PE with and without CIT.

Computed Tomography

CTPA is the imaging study of choice for the diagnosis of PE. It is both sensitive and specific for PE and allows for the assessment of other pulmonary diseases.[22] Although CTPA has allowed for visualization of CIT in isolated case reports,[23,24] it is not an optimal test for the diagnosis of CIT. The timing of the contrast bolus for CTPA is not ideal for imaging of the right heart, and a clot that is isodense with blood flowing through the heart may not be seen. CTPA also does not typically use electrocardiographic gating to minimize artifact due to cardiac motion. In addition, CTPA provides a static image of a highly dynamic process and does not provide assessment of thrombus mobility. CTPA is typically performed only once, so serial assessment of the CIT and its response to treatment are not possible.[24] Last, CTPA may require the removal of an unstable patient from the resuscitation bay.[18] Thus, although CTPA can be helpful identifying additional clot in the pulmonary arteries, it is not useful for diagnosing CIT and should be performed only after a patient with suspected CIT has been stabilized.[3]

Pulmonary Angiography

Catheter pulmonary angiography carries many of the same limitations as CTPA, but is further limited by availability, expertise, and potential complications of catheter placement. Although catheter pulmonary angiography has been used to confirm a CIT diagnosis, catheter placement and contrast injection into the right heart may promote embolization of the CIT.[5] Injecting contrast into the superior vena cava, rather than right heart, may mitigate the risk of dislodging the CIT.[25] However, in one report, this approach was not associated with a change in clinical management.[25] Therefore, the diagnostic role of catheter pulmonary angiography is limited, although it may provide supplementary information in the setting of catheter-based treatment.[3]

Echocardiography

Echocardiography is the imaging modality of choice for the diagnosis and assessment of CIT. Echocardiography can both identify the presence of CIT and can be used to assess acute right ventricular dysfunction, both of which are associated with adverse outcomes in patients with PE.[26] Importantly, echocardiography provides dynamic visualization of mobile thrombi. Thus, echocardiography possesses both diagnostic and prognostic utility for CIT.

Transthoracic echocardiography (TTE) is preferred as the initial imaging modality for several reasons. It is noninvasive, readily available, and can rapidly be performed by trained practitioners who are not formal echocardiographers.[3,16,18,27–30] This allows for rapid diagnosis and initiation of treatment. Furthermore, TTE can be performed at the bedside, which allows the patient to remain in the resuscitation bay. This is particularly important for patients with CIT who often present with compromised, or unpredictable, hemodynamics.[18] Last, clinicians can easily perform serial TTE examinations to monitor the patient's status and the CIT's response to treatment.[9,30,31]

The main limitation of TTE is low sensitivity. Compared with transesophageal echocardiography (TEE), TTE is only 50% to 60% sensitive for the detection of CIT.[32] Therefore, TEE should be strongly considered when concern for CIT is high but TTE is negative or nondiagnostic.[16] In addition to better sensitivity, TEE allows for better visualization of atrial septal abnormalities and is useful if there is concern for CIT crossing a patent foramen ovale (PFO).[33] TEE also can be beneficial if the etiology of a visualized intracardiac mass is unclear. TEE can differentiate CIT from structures such as Chiari networks, Eustachian or Thebesian valves, atrial septal aneurysms, tumors, devices, or vegetations.[3] TEE is also useful for visualizing clots in the main pulmonary arteries and can be used to estimate clot size, which may be helpful in assessing the response to treatment.[3,20] However, TEE is more invasive, less readily available, can delay treatment, and the need for sedation or endotracheal intubation may place hemodynamically compromised patients at risk for decompensation.[3,16,34] Therefore, TEE should be considered only when the potential benefits of making a definitive diagnosis of CIT outweigh the risks of the procedure.[3,34]

PROGNOSIS

CIT is associated with both more severe PE and higher mortality than PE alone.[9] Studies report that patients with CIT are more likely to have right ventricular dysfunction on echocardiography as well as higher Troponin I and B-type natriuretic peptide levels than patients with PE without CIT.[6,9,10,21] Patients with CIT are also more likely to have hemodynamic instability, with lower blood pressures and higher heart rates, than patients with PE without CIT.[9,10] Signs of right ventricular dysfunction and hemodynamic compromise indicate more severe PE and are associated with higher mortality.[22] Similarly, patients with CIT and (chemical or echocardiographic) signs of right ventricular dysfunction, have increased mortality compared with CIT alone.[6,19,35] However, whether the higher mortality is due to the CIT or the more severe PE it is associated with, is uncertain.[10] Additional studies have reported that hemodynamic compromise, shock index greater than 1, and simplified Pulmonary Embolism Severity Index are associated with higher mortality in patients with CIT.[2,17,35–37] On the other hand, characteristics of the clot itself, such as attachment, mobility, and location, have not been found to be associated with mortality in patients with CIT.[4,17,35]

TREATMENT

There is no clear consensus on the optimal treatment for CIT. Given its rarity, our knowledge is limited to case reports, small case series, and meta-analyses that offer conflicting recommendations.[1–7,9,10,12,13,16–21,23–25,27,29–31,33–35] One meta-analysis by Kinney and Wright[4] reported slightly higher survival when patients were treated with anticoagulation alone, compared with systemic thrombolysis or surgical embolectomy. However, another review by Rose and colleagues[5] found systemic thrombolysis to be associated with reduced mortality compared with anticoagulation alone and surgical embolectomy. In contrast, the European Society of Echocardiography reports mortality to be lowest in patients treated with surgical embolectomy.[11] Of course, the potential for publication bias limits the interpretation of each of these reviews and meta-analyses. Given this lack of consensus in the literature and the lack of any randomized control trials, the optimal therapy for CIT is not well established.

Anticoagulation

The European Society of Cardiology (ESC) guidelines recommend empiric parenteral anticoagulation in patients with intermediate and high clinical probability PE, who do not possess absolute contraindications and for whom the bleeding risk is low-moderate, as well as for patients diagnosed with a PE.[26] By extension, therapeutic anticoagulation is recommended in the acute phase for patients with CIT as well.[31,38] In particular, intravenous (IV) unfractionated heparin (UFH) is recommended for patients who may require primary reperfusion, mostly due to the ability to discontinue the infusion and reverse anticoagulation if needed for surgery or other invasive procedures.[26] Case reports have documented success treating patients with IV heparin, particularly in patients with contraindications to thrombolysis or surgery.[31,39,40] Successful treatment with low molecular weight heparin (LMWH) has also been described in a patient who declined thrombolysis or surgery.[41] However, for patients in whom more aggressive treatment is an option, anticoagulation alone seems to be associated with higher mortality compared with thrombolysis and surgical embolectomy, and anticoagulation may increase the risk of distal embolization of the CIT.[16,30,31]

Systemic Thrombolysis

Guidelines state that patients diagnosed with intermediate or high-risk PE may benefit from systemic thrombolysis, although definitive recommendations are not available for CIT.[26] Systemic thrombolysis has the advantage of being administered at the bedside and can dissolve thrombus in the right heart, pulmonary artery, and deep veins simultaneously.[8,30] However, the risk of bleeding, especially intracranial hemorrhage, is high with full-dose systemic thrombolysis. Therefore, in patients with CIT and signs of right ventricular dysfunction or hemodynamic compromise, thrombolysis is a reasonable treatment choice, as long as the risk of bleeding is low. It is possible that bleeding risk can be mitigated by using lower doses of thrombolytic, as described by Patel and colleagues,[42,43] who successfully treated a patient with CIT who had contraindications to thrombolysis with low-dose tissue plasminogen activator, as described in The Moderate Pulmonary Embolism Treated with Thrombolysis (MOPPET) trial. However, because dissolution of thrombus can be uneven, there is always a risk of embolization of the CIT.[8,30,32] This is particularly precarious when CITs cross to the left side of the heart (eg, CIT lodged in a PFO), as lysis can lead to catastrophic paradoxic embolization. In such cases, systemic thrombolysis is not recommended.[16,44]

Surgical Embolectomy

Surgical embolectomy is another option to be considered in the treatment of intermediate and high-risk PE according to ESC guidelines.[26] In particular, emergent surgical embolectomy is recommended for patients with a CIT entrapped in a PFO, given the impending risk of systemic embolization and the opportunity to simultaneously repair the PFO. Surgical embolectomy is also a potential treatment for patients with contraindications to thrombolysis or for whom thrombolysis was ineffective.[8,44] A study by Ferrari and colleagues[9] showed that 50% of CITs treated with thrombolytics disappeared by 2 hours posttreatment whereas an additional 25% disappeared by 12 hours and the remaining 25% disappeared by 24 hours. This delay in thrombus disappearance suggests that health care teams should wait at least 24 hours for thrombolysis to take effect before resorting to surgery.[31] As with any procedure, outcomes of surgical embolectomy are dependent on local expertise, and the relative risk of delayed definitive therapy should be considered, particularly for unstable patients who present to institutions that lack cardiothoracic surgery services where transfer to another facility for surgery would be required. In addition, the risks of cardiopulmonary bypass and general anesthesia in a patient with increased right ventricular pressures needs to be considered. Last, the inability to remove concurrent PE distal to the central pulmonary arteries may limit the procedure's effectiveness.[5,31,45]

Catheter-Based Intervention

Percutaneous catheter-based interventions offer promising alternatives for patients in whom systemic thrombolysis or surgical embolectomy are contraindicated or would not be tolerated. These less-invasive procedures also may be attractive for patients in whom systemic thrombolysis has been ineffective, when the bleeding risk of surgery is unacceptably high.[44] Several successful percutaneous catheter-based interventions have been described in the treatment of CIT, including mechanical fragmentation with a pigtail catheter, basket retrieval, aspiration thrombectomy, and catheter-directed thrombolysis with or without ultrasound assistance.[45–50] However, apart from isolated case reports, our understanding of the effectiveness of catheter-based treatment of CIT is very limited and no comparative data or clinical trials exist. Moreover, there is a theoretic risk of disrupting a CIT with the placement of a catheter in the heart.

OUTCOMES

The overall mortality rate for CIT has been shown to be as high as 45%, and most studies report mortalities between 19% and 38%.[2–4,7,17,19–21,35] Patients with CIT have both a significantly higher short-term all-cause mortality and PE-related mortality than patients with PE without CIT.[1,35] The higher mortality is most apparent when comparing hemodynamically stable patients. Barrios and colleagues[6] found that CIT was associated with higher 30-day all-cause mortality among low-risk patients with PE (odds ratio [OR] 6.71) and intermediate-risk (submassive) patients with PE (OR 2.62), but not among high-risk (massive) patients with PE (OR 1.03). Similarly, Casazza and colleagues[7] did not see a difference in mortality comparing patients with massive PE with CIT (30%) with patients with massive PE without CIT (24%). It is possible that CIT does not increase the already high mortality rate associated with massive PE.[51] However, some studies that exclude hemodynamically unstable patients or adjust for hemodynamic status in propensity-matched analyses, do find that CIT is associated with higher all-cause and PE-related mortality than PE alone.[17,35]

Summary and Future Directions

CIT represents an uncommon, but life-threatening emergency and high-risk form of VTE with mortality as high as 45%.[3] Risk factors for CIT are not well described, but CHF seems to be associated. Patients with CIT are more likely to present with signs of severe PE, so the presence of severe PE, especially in a patient with CHF, should alert physicians to the possibility of CIT. TTE is the first-line diagnostic test, although TEE may ultimately provide more diagnostic information. With conflicting reports in the literature and the lack of any prospective randomized controlled trials, the optimal therapy for CIT is uncertain. However, given the infrequency of CIT, the complexity of this patient population, and institutional differences, the development and validation of a one-size-fits-all treatment algorithm is unlikely.[12,31] Therefore, we advocate for the involvement of multidisciplinary Pulmonary Embolism Response Teams to facilitate the rapid assessment of these patients and to make treatment recommendations based on individual patient factors, institutional resources, and the evolving literature.[12,17,52]

INCIDENTAL PULMONARY EMBOLISM
Introduction

IPE is a challenging clinical problem. There is a dearth of data on how to manage these patients. Current treatment strategies are based on what is done for patients with symptomatic PE. Clinical trials are needed to help clarify the risk-benefit ratio of anticoagulant therapy in patients with IPE.

Definition and Incidence

IPE, also described as "unsuspected PE" or "silent PE," is defined as a filling defect in one or more of the pulmonary arteries seen on imaging that is performed for an indication other than suspected PE. With new advances in computed tomography (CT) technology, and in particular, with the adoption of multiple detector computed tomography scans capable of thinner slices, as well as the increased use of these more advanced imaging modalities, the detection of IPE is increasing. The exact prevalence of IPE is unknown, and it varies among different patient populations. For example, in a large meta-analysis of 12 studies including more than 10,000 patients, the overall prevalence of IPE was 2.6%. However, the prevalence was significantly higher in patients with high-risk VTE factors such as cancer (3.1%) or inpatient status (4.0%).[53] Similarly, in a recent pooled analysis, the weighted frequency of IPE identified on multislice coronary CT scans of 7019 patients from 4 studies was 1.1%, whereas it was 3.6% in a pooled analysis of 8491 patients with cancer from 8 studies involving oncology staging CT scans.[54] Trauma patients have an even higher frequency of IPE. One study found that asymptomatic PE occurred in 24% (95% confidence interval [CI] 16–35) of moderately to severely injured patients, and 30% of patients who received pharmacologic prophylaxis had a PE.[55]

Although the term IPE implies no symptoms, in a retrospective chart review of 46 patients with cancer with an unsuspected PE (UPE) or IPE and 92 matched controls, 75% of the patients had at least 1 symptom suggestive of PE. The patients with PE were also significantly more likely than the control patients to complain of fatigue (54% vs 20%; $P = .0002$) and shortness of breath (22% vs 8%; $P = .02$).[56] In an updated analysis of this study with 70 patients and 137 controls, shortness of breath and fatigue remained significantly more prevalent among the IPE cases than controls, and cough was added to the list of symptoms associated with UPE (16% vs 5%, $P = .019$).[57] In these studies, it is hard to know if the symptoms experienced by the patients with cancer were due to the IPE, the cancer itself, or the cancer treatments. Thus, it is important when evaluating patients for IPE to ask about specific clinical symptoms, as this may have implications for treatment (see **Fig. 1**).

Further Workup

When an IPE is identified, providers should first and foremost carefully review the CT images with a radiologist to confirm the diagnosis. In patients with isolated subsegmental PE, compression ultrasonography of the lower limbs is often recommended to detect the presence of a concomitant incidental DVT and ascertain the degree of clot burden, as this may have implications for treatment (**Fig. 2**) and refer to the algorithm for evaluating Incidental PE. In one study, patients who presented with a first episode of an acute, symptomatic PE, the presence of a concomitant DVT was associated with higher all-cause mortality (adjusted hazard ratio [HR] 2.05; 95% CI 1.24–3.38; $P = .005$) and PE-specific mortality (adjusted HR 4.25; 95% CI 1.61–11.25; $P = .04$) at 3 months.[58] Although the use of lower extremity compression ultrasound has not been specifically evaluated in patients with IPE, extrapolating from these data suggests that assessing the thrombotic burden in patients with IPE may help with risk stratification.

Treatment

Indications

The management of patients with IPE can be a challenge for clinicians, as there are limited data on the treatment or prognostic studies assessing outcomes. There are

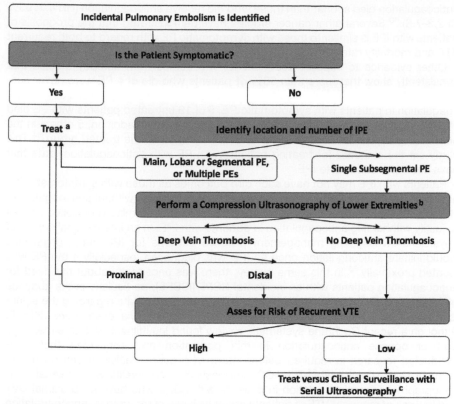

Fig. 2. Workup and treatment for IPE. [a] Please refer to article for anticoagulation treatment options. [b] If patients have a central venous catheter, clinicians should also perform compression ultrasonography of the upper extremities to evaluate for DVT. [c] The decision to treat versus clinical surveillance should be made for each patient by balancing the risks of recurrent VTE with the risks of bleeding, as well as the performance status and preference of each patient.

currently no randomized controlled trials in patients with IPE and, thus, most data come from observational and retrospective studies, most of which involve cancer-associated IPE. As a result, recommendations for the treatment of IPE come primarily from expert opinion. Current consensus, as well as the American College of Chest Physician (ACCP) guidelines advise that IPE should be treated the same as symptomatic PE, as they seem to carry a similar prognosis.

In a recent pooled analysis of 926 patients with cancer with IPE, the 6-month risk of recurrent VTE in patients who were untreated was 12% versus 6.2% and 6.4% in those who were treated with either LMWH or vitamin K antagonist (VKA), respectively.[59] Furthermore, the mortality rate was 47% in the untreated population versus 37% and 28% in those treated with LMWH and VKA, respectively. Importantly, the VTE recurrence risk was comparable in patients with a subsegmental PE (SSPE, PE confined to the subsegmental pulmonary arteries) and those with more proximally localized IPE (HR 1.1; 95% CI 0.50–2.4). This suggests that the risk of recurrence is related more to the risk factors that led to the PE than to the severity of the first PE event. A retrospective observational study that was not included in the aforementioned meta-analysis found that patients with lung cancer with IPE who did not receive anticoagulation died sooner than those who did receive anticoagulation (HR 4.1; 95% CI 2.3–7.6).[60] Several other cancer studies have demonstrated that the prognosis of patients with IPE is similar to those with symptomatic PE with regard to both recurrent VTE and mortality rates.

Other evidence to support treatment for IPE comes from autopsy studies that consistently show that more than 50% of patients who die of a PE were never suspected of having one.[61–63] In one of the earliest studies evaluating the efficacy of anticoagulation in patients with symptomatic PE, 5 of 19 untreated patients with PE died of their PE, whereas none of the 16 treated patients died. In addition, 5 others in the untreated group had a nonfatal recurrence versus none in the treated group.[64] This study set the standard for treating patients with PE with anticoagulation, data that have been extrapolated to IPE.

Patients with IPE may not have such dire outcomes as those with symptomatic PE, and there is even a possibility that IPE may resolve on its own without anticoagulation. However, there are currently no adequately powered or randomized controlled studies to justify withholding anticoagulation in patients with IPE. In an international survey of physicians investigating management practice patterns for IPE, most physicians would initiate anticoagulation once an IPE was diagnosed, especially if the PE was located proximally.[65] In this same survey, there was uncertainty about the need for anticoagulating patients with an incidental SSPE (ISSPE), particularly in the absence of cancer or DVT.[65] This uncertainty stems from conflicting data regarding the significance of ISSPE, which in turn, makes treatment decisions even more difficult. Although a recent Cochrane systematic review found insufficient data to either support or oppose anticoagulation in this population and concluded that well-conducted research is required before informed practice decisions can be made, some guidance does exist.[66] The ACCP suggests clinical surveillance and serial ultrasonography over anticoagulation in patients with SSPE who have no proximal DVT and low risk of recurrent VTE. If patients are at high risk of recurrence, anticoagulation over clinical surveillance is suggested.[67] Similarly, the International Society of Thrombosis and Hemostasis recommends that in patients with ISSPE, the decision to anticoagulate should be made on an individual basis and should consider the risks of bleeding and the persistence of VTE risk factors, in addition to the performance status and preference of the patient.[68] If the decision is not to anticoagulate and the patient has distal DVT, serial compression ultrasonography is recommended (see **Fig. 1**).

If there is a subset of patients with PE who do not need to be treated, this could translate into an economic benefit as well as an overall health benefit for the patient. Fortunately, there is an ongoing trial evaluating the safety of withholding anticoagulation in patients with ISSPE who have no evidence of DVT. This trial is important because, in addition to the potential bleeding risks associated with anticoagulants, there is considerable cost connected with anticoagulant medications and associated health care resources. Annual incident (first) VTE events cost the US health care system $7 to 10 billion each year for 375,000 to 425,000 newly diagnosed, medically treated incident VTE cases.[69] Even with these large numbers, the optimal management of patients with IPE has not been adequately addressed and remains a subject of debate. Ultimately, the decision to initiate anticoagulant therapy in patients with IPE must be based on the risks and benefits of treatment, but also patient preferences, quality of life, and cost.

Anticoagulant agents

The type and duration of anticoagulation for the treatment of IPE is similar to those who present with symptomatic PE. The choice of anticoagulant depends on several factors including patient-related factors (comorbidities, bleeding risks, adherence be-haviors, preferences, medications, and weight), medication-related factors (properties of the drugs and potential drug-drug interactions), and clinical judgment. An additional deciding factor, and one that is often the most influential, is what medication is covered by the patient's insurance. Up until this decade, the only oral anticoagulant for the treatment and prevention of PE approved by the Food and Drug Administration was the VKA, warfarin. The direct oral anticoagulants (DOACs), which include the fac-tor Xa inhibitors apixaban (Eliquis), rivaroxaban (Xarelto), and edoxaban (Savaysa), as well as the factor II or direct thrombin inhibitor dabigatran (Pradaxa), now offer patients an alternative to warfarin. These DOACs represent a major advancement in the treat-ment of PE because they have rapid onset of action, minimal drug interactions, decreased bleeding risk, and comparable efficacy to VKA. They are all currently approved for the treatment and secondary prevention of VTE.

Akin to symptomatic PE, the treatment strategy for treating IPE is divided into 3 phases: acute (the first 5–10 days), short-term (3–6 months), and long-term (>6 months). During the acute setting, anticoagulation options include UFH, LMWH, fondaparinux, rivaroxaban, or apixaban. Dabigatran and edoxaban are effective DOACs as well, but both require 5 to 10 days of an initial parenteral anticoagulant and neither are approved for stand-alone therapy initially. The short-term and long-term anticoagulation options include DOAC and VKA with the former being preferred in most populations because of their superior safety profile and convenience.

Importantly, there are some populations in which DOACs are either not recommen-ded (eg, antiphospholipid syndrome, liver or renal failure) or in whom their efficacy and safety is unknown. For example, until recently, the standard of care for cancer-associated thromboembolism (CAT) was LMWH. However, 2 recent randomized controlled trials in CAT demonstrated that, at least in the short term, edoxaban and rivaroxaban seem as effective as the LMWH, dalteparin.[70,71] However, both DOACs were associated with an increased risk of bleeding when compared with dalteparin, and this bleeding was primarily seen in patients with gastrointestinal tumors. There is an ongoing trial of apixaban and LMWH in patients with cancer. Whether one of these DOACs is superior to another is currently unknown. Thus, given this recent data, clinicians should carefully review the pros (decreased risk of VTE) and cons (increased risk of bleeding) surrounding the use of rivaroxaban and edoxaban in pa-tients with cancer with IPE and decide which anticoagulant to use through a shared decision-making process.

Length of anticoagulation

Similar to treating patients with symptomatic PE, the length of anticoagulation for IPE will depend on the presence or resolution of the patient's thrombotic risk factors. For patients in whom a transient risk has resolved, short-term (eg, 3 month) therapy may be reasonable. Alternatively, for patients with an unprovoked IPE or those with a pro-voked IPE with ongoing risk factors, long-term or even lifelong anticoagulation may be warranted.[67,72–74] Ultimately, the decision regarding the duration of anticoagulation should be individualized for each patient and should include the initial and periodic assessment of risk factors for recurrent PE, balanced against risk factors for bleeding on anticoagulation. Overall, this risk/benefit appraisal should also include patient preference.

Summary and Future Directions

With new advances and increased use of CT imaging, the diagnosis of IPE is increasing. Although there are very few studies that highlight the natural course of

IPE, consensus is that the prognosis is similar to that of symptomatic PE in terms of recurrent PE and mortality. As such, current guidelines suggest that patients with IPE should be treated similar to those with symptomatic PE. Large randomized controlled trials investigating the optimal management and outcomes of IPE are much needed, and a few are presently under way.

SUMMARY

CIT and IPE are 2 complex situations faced by clinicians treating patients with PE. In both situations, the clinical severity of symptoms may not correlate with the thrombus burden or the potential risk to the patient. Although robust data that define the optimal approach to either of these situations are sparse, the data that are available can provide some guidance to clinicians as they manage patients with PE across the clinical severity spectrum.

REFERENCES

1. Barrios D, Rosa-Salazar V, Morillo R, et al. Prognostic significance of right heart thrombi in patients with acute symptomatic pulmonary embolism: systematic review and meta-analysis. Chest 2017;151(2):409–16.
2. Athappan G, Sengodan P, Chacko P, et al. Comparative efficacy of different modalities for treatment of right heart thrombi in transit: a pooled analysis. Vasc Med 2015;20(2):131–8.
3. Chartier L, Bera J, Delomez M, et al. Free-floating thrombi in the right heart: diagnosis, management, and prognostic indexes in 38 consecutive patients. Circulation 1999;99(21):2779–83.
4. Kinney EL, Wright RJ. Efficacy of treatment of patients with echocardiographically detected right-sided heart thrombi: a meta-analysis. Am Heart J 1989;118(3):569–73.
5. Rose PS, Punjabi NM, Pearse DB. Treatment of right heart thromboemboli. Chest 2002;121(3):806–14.
6. Barrios D, Rosa-Salazar V, Jimenez D, et al. Right heart thrombi in pulmonary embolism. Eur Respir J 2016;48(5):1377–85.
7. Casazza F, Bongarzoni A, Centonze F, et al. Prevalence and prognostic significance of right-sided cardiac mobile thrombi in acute massive pulmonary embolism. Am J Cardiol 1997;79(10):1433–5.
8. Nkoke C, Faucher O, Camus L, et al. Free floating right heart thrombus associated with acute pulmonary embolism: an unsettled therapeutic difficulty. Case Rep Cardiol 2015;2015:364780.
9. Ferrari E, Benhamou M, Berthier F, et al. Mobile thrombi of the right heart in pulmonary embolism: delayed disappearance after thrombolytic treatment. Chest 2005;127(3):1051–3.
10. Torbicki A, Galie N, Covezzoli A, et al. Right heart thrombi in pulmonary embolism: results from the International Cooperative Pulmonary Embolism Registry. J Am Coll Cardiol 2003;41(12):2245–51.
11. The European Cooperative Study on the clinical significance of right heart thrombi. European Working Group on Echocardiography. Eur Heart J 1989;10(12):1046–59.
12. Pappas AJ, Knight SW, McLean KZ, et al. Thrombus-in-transit: a case for a multidisciplinary hospital-based pulmonary embolism system of care. J Emerg Med 2016;51(3):298–302.

13. Farfel Z, Shechter M, Vered Z, et al. Review of echocardiographically diagnosed right heart entrapment of pulmonary emboli-in-transit with emphasis on management. Am Heart J 1987;113(1):171–8.

14. Bagot CN, Arya R. Virchow and his triad: a question of attribution. Br J Haematol 2008;143(2):180–90.

15. Spencer FA, Emery C, Lessard D, et al. The Worcester Venous Thromboembolism study: a population-based study of the clinical epidemiology of venous thromboembolism. J Gen Intern Med 2006;21(7):722–7.

16. Agarwal V, Nalluri N, Shariff MA, et al. Large embolus in transit - an unresolved therapeutic dilemma (case report and review of literature). Heart Lung 2014; 43(2):152–4.

17. Islam M, Nesheim D, Acquah S, et al. Right heart thrombi: patient outcomes by treatment modality and predictors of mortality: a pooled analysis. J Intensive Care Med 2018. [Epub ahead of print].

18. Fischer JI, Huis in 't Veld MA, Orland M, et al. Diagnosis of near-fatal pulmonary embolus-in-transit with focused echocardiography. J Emerg Med 2013;45(2): 232–5.

19. Akilli H, Gul EE, Aribas A, et al. Management of right heart thrombi associated with acute pulmonary embolism: a retrospective, single-center experience. Anadolu Kardiyol Derg 2013;13(6):528–33.

20. Burgos LM, Costabel JP, Galizia Brito V, et al. Floating right heart thrombi: a pooled analysis of cases reported over the past 10 years. Am J Emerg Med 2018;36(6):911–5.

21. Mollazadeh R, Ostovan MA, Abdi Ardekani AR. Right cardiac thrombus in transit among patients with pulmonary thromboemboli. Clin Cardiol 2009;32(6):E27–31.

22. Stein PD, Beemath A, Matta F, et al. Clinical characteristics of patients with acute pulmonary embolism: data from PIOPED II. Am J Med 2007;120(10):871–9.

23. Kabrhel C, Rempell JS, Avery LL, et al. Case records of the Massachusetts General Hospital. Case 29-2014. A 60-year-old woman with syncope. N Engl J Med 2014;371(12):1143–50.

24. Leach JR, Elicker B, Yee J, et al. Clot through the heart: paradoxical embolism with thrombus-in-transit at multidetector computed tomography. J Comput Assist Tomogr 2015;39(4):598–600.

25. Cameron J, Pohlner PG, Stafford EG, et al. Right heart thrombus: recognition, diagnosis and management. J Am Coll Cardiol 1985;5(5):1239–43.

26. Konstantinides SV, Torbicki A, Agnelli G, et al. 2014 ESC guidelines on the diagnosis and management of acute pulmonary embolism. Eur Heart J 2014;35(43): 3033–69, 3069a–3069k.

27. Jammal M, Milano P, Cardenas R, et al. The diagnosis of right heart thrombus by focused cardiac ultrasound in a critically ill patient in compensated shock. Crit Ultrasound J 2015;7:6.

28. Labovitz AJ, Noble VE, Bierig M, et al. Focused cardiac ultrasound in the emergent setting: a consensus statement of the American Society of Echocardiography and American College of Emergency Physicians. J Am Soc Echocardiogr 2010;23(12):1225–30.

29. Martires JS, Stein SJ, Kamangar N. Right heart thrombus in transit diagnosed by bedside ultrasound. J Emerg Med 2015;48(4):e105–8.

30. Naeem K. Floating thrombus in the right heart associated with pulmonary embolism: the role of echocardiography. Pak J Med Sci 2015;31(1):233–5.

31. Portugues J, Calvo L, Oliveira M, et al. Pulmonary embolism and intracardiac type A thrombus with an unexpected outcome. Case Rep Cardiol 2017;2017: 9092576.

32. Obeid AI, al Mudamgha A, Smulyan H. Diagnosis of right atrial mass lesions by transesophageal and transthoracic echocardiography. Chest 1993;103(5): 1447–51.

33. Ellensen VS, Saeed S, Geisner T, et al. Management of thromboembolism-in-transit with pulmonary embolism. Echo Res Pract 2017;4(4):K47–51.

34. Pierre-Justin G, Pierard LA. Management of mobile right heart thrombi: a prospective series. Int J Cardiol 2005;99(3):381–8.

35. Koc M, Kostrubiec M, Elikowski W, et al. Outcome of patients with right heart thrombi: the right heart thrombi European Registry. Eur Respir J 2016;47(3): 869–75.

36. Allgower M, Burri C. Shock index. Dtsch Med Wochenschr 1967;92(43):1947–50 [in German].

37. Jimenez D, Aujesky D, Moores L, et al. Simplification of the pulmonary embolism severity index for prognostication in patients with acute symptomatic pulmonary embolism. Arch Intern Med 2010;170(15):1383–9.

38. Charif F, Mansour MJ, Hamdan R, et al. Free-floating right heart thrombus with acute massive pulmonary embolism: a case report and review of the literature. J Cardiovasc Echogr 2018;28(2):146–9.

39. Hinton JW, Lainchbury J, Crozier I. Right atrial mass–a venous thrombosis in transit. N Z Med J 2012;125(1363):81–3.

40. Temtanakitpaisan Y, Mahatanan R, Rishikof DC, et al. Use of heparin alone in treating pulmonary emboli found in association with in-transit right-heart thrombi in a nonagenarian. Tex Heart Inst J 2013;40(4):487–8.

41. Lampropoulos KM, Bonou M, Theocharis C, et al. Treatment of mobile right heart thrombi with low-molecular-weight heparin. BMJ Case Rep 2013;2013.

42. Patel AK, Kafi A, Bonet A, et al. Resolution of a mobile right atrial thrombus complicating acute pulmonary embolism with low-dose tissue plasminogen activator in a patient with recent craniotomy. J Intensive Care Med 2016;31(9): 618–21.

43. Sharifi M, Bay C, Skrocki L, et al. Moderate pulmonary embolism treated with thrombolysis (from the "MOPETT" Trial). Am J Cardiol 2013;111(2):273–7.

44. Dzudovic B, Obradovic S, Rusovic S, et al. Therapeutic approach in patients with a floating thrombus in the right heart. J Emerg Med 2013;44(2):e199–205.

45. Beregi JP, Aumegeat V, Loubeyre C, et al. Right atrial thrombi: percutaneous mechanical thrombectomy. Cardiovasc Intervent Radiol 1997;20(2):142–5.

46. Davies RP, Harding J, Hassam R. Percutaneous retrieval of a right atrioventricular embolus. Cardiovasc Intervent Radiol 1998;21(5):433–5.

47. Momose T, Morita T, Misawa T. Percutaneous treatment of a free-floating thrombus in the right atrium of a patient with pulmonary embolism and acute myocarditis. Cardiovasc Interv Ther 2013;28(2):188–92.

48. Nickel B, McClure T, Moriarty J. A novel technique for endovascular removal of large volume right atrial tumor thrombus. Cardiovasc Intervent Radiol 2015; 38(4):1021–4.

49. Santos Martinez LE, Uriona Villarroel JE, Exaire Rodriguez JE, et al. Massive pulmonary embolism, thrombus in transit, and right ventricular dysfunction. Arch Cardiol Mex 2007;77(1):44–53 [in Spanish].

50. Shammas NW, Padaria R, Ahuja G. Ultrasound-assisted lysis using recombinant tissue plasminogen activator and the EKOS EkoSonic endovascular system for

treating right atrial thrombus and massive pulmonary embolism: a case study. Phlebology 2015;30(10):739–43.

51. Konstantinov IE, Saxena P, Koniuszko MD, et al. Acute massive pulmonary embolism with cardiopulmonary resuscitation: management and results. Tex Heart Inst J 2007;34(1):41–5 [discussion: 45–6].

52. Kabrhel C, Rosovsky R, Channick R, et al. A multidisciplinary pulmonary embolism response team: initial 30-month experience with a novel approach to delivery of care to patients with submassive and massive pulmonary embolism. Chest 2016;150(2):384–93.

53. Dentali F, Ageno W, Becattini C, et al. Prevalence and clinical history of incidental, asymptomatic pulmonary embolism: a meta-analysis. Thromb Res 2010;125(6): 518–22.

54. Klok FA, Huisman MV. Management of incidental pulmonary embolism. Eur Respir J 2017;49(6).

55. Schultz DJ, Brasel KJ, Washington L, et al. Incidence of asymptomatic pulmonary embolism in moderately to severely injured trauma patients. J Trauma 2004;56(4): 727–31 [discussion: 731–3].

56. O'Connell CL, Boswell WD, Duddalwar V, et al. Unsuspected pulmonary emboli in cancer patients: clinical correlates and relevance. J Clin Oncol 2006;24(30): 4928–32.

57. O'Connell C, Razavi P, Ghalichi M, et al. Unsuspected pulmonary emboli adversely impact survival in patients with cancer undergoing routine staging multi-row detector computed tomography scanning. J Thromb Haemost 2011; 9(2):305–11.

58. Jimenez D, Aujesky D, Diaz G, et al. Prognostic significance of deep vein thrombosis in patients presenting with acute symptomatic pulmonary embolism. Am J Respir Crit Care Med 2010;181(9):983–91.

59. van der Hulle T, den Exter PL, Planquette B, et al. Risk of recurrent venous thromboembolism and major hemorrhage in cancer-associated incidental pulmonary embolism among treated and untreated patients: a pooled analysis of 926 patients. J Thromb Haemost 2016;14(1):105–13.

60. Sun JM, Kim TS, Lee J, et al. Unsuspected pulmonary emboli in lung cancer patients: the impact on survival and the significance of anticoagulation therapy. Lung Cancer 2010;69(3):330–6.

61. Goldhaber SZ, Hennekens CH, Evans DA, et al. Factors associated with correct antemortem diagnosis of major pulmonary embolism. Am J Med 1982;73(6): 822–6.

62. Pineda LA, Hathwar VS, Grant BJ. Clinical suspicion of fatal pulmonary embolism. Chest 2001;120(3):791–5.

63. Rubinstein I, Murray D, Hoffstein V. Fatal pulmonary emboli in hospitalized patients. An autopsy study. Arch Intern Med 1988;148(6):1425–6.

64. Barritt DW, Jordan SC. Anticoagulant drugs in the treatment of pulmonary embolism. A controlled trial. Lancet 1960;1(7138):1309–12.

65. den Exter PL, van Roosmalen MJ, van den Hoven P, et al. Physicians' management approach to an incidental pulmonary embolism: an international survey. J Thromb Haemost 2013;11(1):208–13.

66. Yoo HH, Queluz TH, El Dib R. Anticoagulant treatment for subsegmental pulmonary embolism. Cochrane Database Syst Rev 2014;(4):CD010222.

67. Kearon C, Akl EA, Ornelas J, et al. Antithrombotic therapy for VTE disease: CHEST guideline and expert panel report. Chest 2016;149(2):315–52.

68. Di Nisio M, Lee AY, Carrier M, et al. Diagnosis and treatment of incidental venous thromboembolism in cancer patients: guidance from the SSC of the ISTH. J Thromb Haemost 2015;13(5):880–3.
69. Grosse SD, Nelson RE, Nyarko KA, et al. The economic burden of incident venous thromboembolism in the United States: a review of estimated attributable healthcare costs. Thromb Res 2016;137:3–10.
70. Raskob GE, van Es N, Verhamme P, et al. Edoxaban for the treatment of cancer-associated venous thromboembolism. N Engl J Med 2018;378(7):615–24.
71. Young AM, Marshall A, Thirlwall J, et al. Comparison of an oral factor Xa inhibitor with low molecular weight heparin in patients with cancer with venous thromboembolism: results of a randomized trial (SELECT-D). J Clin Oncol 2018;36(20):2017–23.
72. Agnelli G, Buller HR, Cohen A, et al. Apixaban for extended treatment of venous thromboembolism. N Engl J Med 2013;368(8):699–708.
73. Kearon C, Akl EA, Comerota AJ, et al. Antithrombotic therapy for VTE disease: antithrombotic therapy and prevention of thrombosis, 9th ed: American College of Chest Physicians Evidence-Based Clinical Practice Guidelines. Chest 2012;141(2 Suppl):e419S–94S.
74. Weitz JI, Lensing AWA, Prins MH, et al. Rivaroxaban or aspirin for extended treatment of venous thromboembolism. N Engl J Med 2017;376(13):1211–22.

Pulmonary Embolism in the Intensive Care Unit: Therapy in Subpopulations

John R. Bartholomew, MD, MSVM

KEYWORDS

- Pulmonary embolism • Risk factors for pulmonary embolism during pregnancy and the postpartum state • Diagnosis of pulmonary embolism in the pregnant patient
- Anticoagulation for the pregnant patient
- Advanced therapies for acute submassive or massive pulmonary embolism during pregnancy and the postpartum state
- Placement of an IVC filter in the pregnant patient
- Diagnosis of PE in the cancer patient • Treatment of cancer-associated thrombosis

KEY POINTS

- Confirm the diagnosis of pulmonary embolism in the patient who is pregnant and the patient with cancer.
- Review advanced treatment options for the pregnant and postpartum patient and patient with cancer with submassive or massive acute pulmonary embolism.
- Treatment of cancer-associated pulmonary embolism in the patient with thrombocytopenia.
- Treatment of cancer-associated thrombosis in the bleeding patient.

THE PREGNANT PATIENT

Venous thromboembolism (VTE), which includes deep vein thrombosis (DVT) and pulmonary embolism (PE), is a common complication of pregnancy. Acute PE is one of the leading causes of pregnancy-related maternal deaths in Western countries.[1,2] PE complicates 1 to 2 of every 1000 pregnancies and accounts for approximately 1.5 deaths per 100,000 deliveries.[3] Compared with nonpregnant women, pregnant women have a fourfold higher risk of PE. The risk of PE increases with each trimester and is even higher in the postpartum period, peaking 1 to 3 weeks postpartum and declines to a risk equivalent nonpregnant woman by 12 weeks postpartum.[3]

Vascular Medicine, Department of Cardiovascular Medicine, Cleveland Clinic, 9500 Euclid Avenue J3-5, Cleveland, OH 44195, USA
E-mail address: barthoj@ccf.org

Crit Care Clin 36 (2020) 547–560
https://doi.org/10.1016/j.ccc.2020.03.001   criticalcare.theclinics.com
0749-0704/20/© 2020 Elsevier Inc. All rights reserved.

RISK FACTORS

There are a number of risk factors associated with the development of VTE during pregnancy and the postpartum state. Risk factors are listed in **Table 1** for pregnancy and **Box 1** for the postpartum state.

Table 1
Risk factors for pregnancy-associated venous thromboembolism

Increased Age	Thrombophilia
Immobilization (strict bed rest for a week or more during the antepartum period)	Family history of venous thromboembolism
Body mass index >25 kg/m²	Varicose veins
Smoking (before or during pregnancy)	Inflammatory bowel disease
Preeclampsia	Diabetes mellitus
Cesarean delivery	Hypertension
Multiple pregnancies	Sickle cell anemia

Data from Refs.[4,5]

Box 1
Risk factors for postpartum venous thromboembolism

Age, body mass index, smoking

Diabetes, hypertension, cardiovascular disease, inflammatory bowel disease

Delivery complications: type of delivery (cesarean), stillbirth, preterm birth, postpartum hemorrhage, postpartum infection

Data from Refs.[4–6]

INCIDENCE

Studies using the Nationwide Inpatient Sample (NIS), a large database of all payer US inpatient hospital stays derived from billing data, showed overall increases beginning in the mid-1990s in pregnancy-associated VTE events.[7,8] From 1994 to 2009 there was a 14% increase in the rate of overall VTE pregnancy-related hospitalizations while antepartum and postpartum hospitalizations increased by 17% and 47%, respectively.[8] These increases were largely thought due to a rise in the diagnosis of PE related to the use of computed tomographic pulmonary angiography (CTPA). A recent review by Karon and colleagues[3] reported a decrease in the rates of DVT but pointed out that PE rates have remain unchanged as a cause of maternal mortality.

PATHOPHYSIOLOGY OF PULMONARY EMBOLISM IN THE PREGNANT PATIENT

The pathophysiology of VTE in pregnancy is best explained by the Virchow's triad: venous stasis, vascular damage, and hypercoagulability. Venous stasis results from a decreased rate of venous return due to pelvic venous compression or obstruction by the gravid uterus, pulsatile compression of the left iliac vein by the right iliac artery, and hormonal changes decreasing venous tone.[9,10] Vascular damage can occur to the pelvic vessels as a result of venous distension and compression at normal vaginal or cesarean deliveries, whereas a hypercoagulable state results from an increase in procoagulant factors (fibrinogen, factors V, VIII, IX, and X), a decrease in anticoagulant factors (protein S and activated protein C resistance), and an inhibition in fibrinolytic activity resulting in more thrombin generation and less clot dissolution.[10,11]

DIAGNOSIS

Published reports of pregnant women investigated for suspected PE in the emergency department have shown a prevalence of less than 5% among symptomatic pregnant women compared with a rate of 15% to 20% in nonpregnant women, suggesting emergency room physicians have a low threshold for testing.[12] Clinical prediction scores for VTE may be considered less reliable in pregnancy. The most common presenting signs and symptoms of PE, including shortness of breath, pleuritic chest pain, tachycardia, and leg pain and swelling, also can be present in any pregnant woman, making the diagnosis more difficult. Several differences should be noted, however. The swelling in pregnancy is most likely to be symmetric, unlike a DVT that is usually unilateral. Pregnant women may complain of dyspnea on exertion but this generally recovers with rest, and pleuritic chest pain is uncommon during a normal pregnancy. The presence of pleuritic chest pain along with persistent shortness of breath should lead the clinician to suspect PE.[10]

A normal D-dimer is helpful in excluding the diagnosis of PE during pregnancy; however, D-dimer levels rise throughout gestation and therefore the standard cutoff value of 500 ng/mL may be less useful in pregnancy.

Because the signs and symptoms of PE are nonspecific and the D-dimer has low specificity and sensitivity in pregnancy, most pregnant women with a suspected PE will undergo CTPA or a ventilation-perfusion lung scan (V/Q), both of which involve radiation exposure to the mother and fetus. Recently, Righini and colleagues[13] proposed a diagnostic algorithm based on assessment of clinical probability (using the revised Geneva score), D-dimer, bilateral lower limb compression ultrasound (CUS), and CTPA to safely rule out PE in 395 pregnant women. PE was excluded in patients with a low or intermediate pretest clinical probability and a negative D-dimer. All other underwent CUS and if negative a CTPA. Pulmonary embolism was diagnosed in 28 and proximal DVT in 7 women, respectively. The 3-month rate of symptomatic VTE was 0.0% among untreated women and met the proposed criteria by the International Society on Thrombosis and Haemostasis (ISTH) for confirming the safety of this VTE diagnostic strategy.[14]

van der Pol and colleagues[15] assessed 3 criteria from the YEARS algorithm (clinical signs of DVT, hemoptysis, and PE as the most likely diagnosis) and measured D-dimer levels. If the D-dimer level was less than 1000 ng/mL and none of the 3 criteria was present, PE was excluded. If 1 or more of the 3 criteria were met and the D-dimer was less than 500 ng/mL, PE also was excluded. CUS was used with the YEARS algorithm if symptoms of DVT were present. In their study of 510 women screened using this approach (12 were excluded), PE was diagnosed in 20 patients and 1 had a popliteal DVT. Using the pregnancy-adapted YEARS diagnostic algorithm, CTPA was avoided in 32% to 65% of patients depending on their trimester of presentation without compromising safety.[15]

IMAGING

A correct diagnosis is essential because missing a PE can be fatal. Avoiding overdiagnosis is equally important because of long-term implications including the risk of bleeding during delivery, requirement of thromboprophylaxis during future pregnancies, and withholding estrogen contraception.[1] It is reasonable in pregnant women with a suspicion for PE to start with CUS because a positive scan can avoid additional imaging and treatment for DVT is the same as for PE in most patients. CUS assay is also readily available and avoids radiation. If there is no DVT, radiological imaging using either a CTPA or V/Q scan will need to be performed. Using modern imaging techniques, maternal and fetal radiation exposure are very low, and avoiding imaging based on maternal cancer risk or fetal radiation complications is not justified.[1]

If the patient is hemodynamically unstable, CTPA is the preferred first test. It can rule out other life-threatening diagnoses that mimic PE. An algorithm for the diagnosis of a suspected PE in pregnancy is shown in **Fig. 1**.[16]

Other imaging, including magnetic resonance angiography, has shown value in the detection of DVT but has not been validated and not currently recommended for the diagnosis of PE. It requires gadolinium, and the long-term effects on the fetus are not known.

Newer modalities, including the V/Q single-photon emission computed tomography imaging, have shown promise in diagnosing PE in pregnancy with low fetal and maternal radiation exposure, but further evaluation is required.[1]

TREATMENT

Unfractionated heparin and low molecular weight heparin (LMWH) are used for the treatment of VTE in pregnancy because they do not cross the placenta and pose little risk of fetal hemorrhage or teratogenicity. LMWH is the treatment of choice because it has reliable pharmacokinetics and the dose has a linear relationship to anti-XA activity. There is also a lower incidence of heparin-induced thrombocytopenia (HIT), less risk for osteoporosis compared with heparin, and bleeding risk is low. Dosing is similar to nonpregnant women and monitoring using plasma anti-activated coagulation factor X activity levels is not generally recommended unless the patient has extremes of body weight or renal disease.[1]

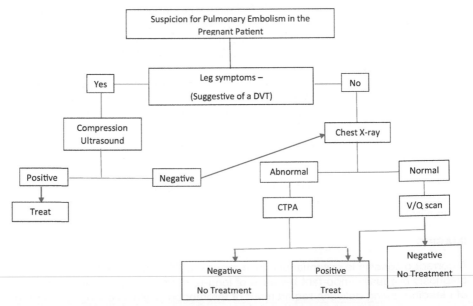

Fig. 1. Suggested algorithm for the diagnosis of PE in the pregnant patient.

Fondaparinux has been used in patients allergic to heparin or LMWH. A review of maternal outcomes of 65 patients found it well tolerated during pregnancy with complication rates similar to the general population.[17] It crosses the placenta in small quantities with no documented fetal consequences.[10]

Vitamin K antagonists cross the placenta and are associated with embryopathy during the first trimester as well as central nervous system anomalies and are not recommended for use in the United States.

There are no data on the direct oral anticoagulants (DOACs), as pregnant women were excluded from clinical trials. In accordance with the European Society of Cardiology (ESC) guidelines, DOACs are contraindicated during pregnancy.[1]

ADVANCED THERAPIES

PE is one of the most common causes of cardiovascular collapse in pregnant women.[18] The optimal management of a submassive or massive PE during pregnancy is unclear because of a lack of large clinical trials. Evaluation of the patient who may be a candidate for more aggressive therapy includes the use of biomarkers and echocardiogram for risk stratification. Both brain natriuretic peptides (BNPs) or N-terminal (NT)-proBNP suggest right ventricular pressure overload and help determine if a more aggressive approach to the patient's management should be considered. Elevated troponin levels at the time of admission are helpful as well, and suggest a worse prognosis.[1] Demonstration of right ventricle overload and dysfunction on echocardiogram is also useful as well for risk stratification of the disease.

For the hemodynamically unstable pregnant patient at high risk for death or the patient at intermediate risk with abnormal biomarkers or right ventricular dysfunction, treatment options include thrombolysis (systemic or catheter-directed therapy), percutaneous catheter-based mechanical thrombectomy, surgical embolectomy, or placement of an inferior vena cava (IVC) filter if anticoagulation is contraindicated.

SYSTEMIC THROMBOLYSIS

Thrombolysis had once been considered a contraindication during pregnancy and the postpartum state. Ahearn and colleagues[19] successfully treated a patient with a massive PE during pregnancy using recombinant tissue plasminogen activator (rt-PA) (**Fig. 2**). In their case report and review of the literature involving nearly 200 patients who received thrombolytic therapy (most were not PE) during their 14th to 40th week of pregnancy, maternal mortality rates of 1%, fetal loss of 6%, and premature delivery of 6% were reported.[19] Most patients were treated with streptokinase with only 3 receiving urokinase and 5 rt-PA. They concluded that thrombolytic therapy was safe with low maternal and fetal mortality rates.[19]

Leonhardt and colleagues[20] reviewed 28 cases of pregnant women receiving systemic thrombolysis (7 PEs), most received 100 mg of rt-PA over 2 hours. No maternal deaths, 1 fetal death, and 1 spontaneous abortion were reported. The investigators noted that thrombolysis complication rates did not exceed those of large randomized controlled trials for the general population with VTE and concluded thrombolytic therapy should not be withheld in pregnant patients in cases of life-threatening or potentially debilitating thromboembolic disease.

Thirteen cases of massive PE reported by te Raa and colleagues[21] were successfully treated with thrombolytic therapy in their review of the literature. No maternal deaths, 2 fetal deaths, and 5 preterm deliveries were described, and these investigators similarly concluded withholding thrombolytic therapy was not justified in cases of life-threatening PE during pregnancy.[21]

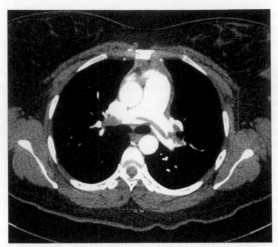

Fig. 2. A 25-year-old woman in her third trimester presented with shortness of breath, pleuritic chest pain, and tachycardia. Her risk factors included elevated body mass index, hypertension, diabetes, and smoking history before her pregnancy. She was hypotensive, had elevated biomarkers and right ventricular dysfunction on echocardiogram (not shown), and received rt-PA without complications.

A recent systematic review by Martillotti and colleagues[22] described 127 cases of severe high-risk and intermediate-risk PE during pregnancy and 6 weeks postpartum treated with thrombolysis, percutaneous or mechanical thrombectomy, and/or extracorporeal membrane oxygenation (ECMO). Survival rates of women receiving thrombolysis were 94% and 88% during pregnancy and postpartum, respectively, with major bleeding rates of 17.5% during pregnancy and 58.3% postpartum, respectively. There was a 12% incidence of fetal death possibly related to bleeding or PE.[22] Approximately one-half of postpartum PE occurred within 24 hours of delivery. The investigators concluded that evidence supported the use of thrombolytic therapy for acute PE both during pregnancy and postpartum.[22]

Potential complications of systemic thrombolysis include intracranial hemorrhage, maternal hemorrhage, preterm delivery, fetal loss, spontaneous abortion, vaginal bleeding, uterine bleeding requiring emergency cesarean delivery, and postpartum hemorrhage requiring transfusion.[23]

Of note, the recent ESC guidelines advise that thrombolytic therapy should not be used peripartum except in the setting of life-threatening PE.[1]

CATHETER-DIRECTED THERAPIES

There are few data on catheter-directed (CDT) thrombolytic therapy during pregnancy or postpartum. te Raa and colleagues[21] reviewed results of CDT, including mechanical embolectomy and thrombolytic therapy. Of 4 reported cases, 2 received rt-PA preceded by mechanical embolectomy, 1 urokinase, and 1 mechanical embolectomy alone. There was 1 fetal death and 1 preterm delivery. The investigators advised that CDT be performed only at centers with appropriate facilities and expertise.[21]

Martillotti and colleagues[22] reviewed 7 cases of severe PE (6 massive) that received percutaneous fragmentation or thromboaspiration without thrombolysis. Two of the patients required ECMO, but the maternal survival rate was 100%. Major bleeding was 20% and fetal death rate 25%.

SURGICAL EMBOLECTOMY

Surgical embolectomy is an option if there is a contraindication to thrombolytic therapy or if conventional therapy or thrombolysis fails. It should be performed only at centers with facilities for cardiopulmonary bypass and experienced surgeons. There are few published data on surgical embolectomy and outcomes for PE in pregnancy. te Raa and colleagues[21] described 8 cases of massive PE that had surgical embolectomy. There were no maternal deaths, 3 fetal deaths, and 4 preterm deliveries. Maternal survival was acceptable, but fetal death rate was substantial.

In a more recent review, Fukuda and colleagues[24] reported results of 3 cases of pulmonary embolectomy (**Fig. 3**). Two of the 3 underwent cesarean delivery at 28 and 29 weeks. There were no maternal deaths but 1 fetal death during surgery.

Martillotti and colleagues[22] reviewed 36 patients with surgical embolectomy and included 13 who had cardiac arrest. Seven of the women had an emergency cesarean delivery before surgical embolectomy, and 3 had embolectomy after percutaneous fragmentation or thrombolysis. Maternal survival was 86% for surgical embolectomy. Two deaths occurred shortly after or during surgery, major bleeding was 20% and fetal deaths were 20%. Martillotti and colleagues[22] recommended percutaneous or surgical embolectomy or ECMO following delivery because of the high risk of postpartum bleeding with thrombolysis.

EXTRACORPOREAL MEMBRANE OXYGENATION

There are limited data on the use of ECMO during pregnancy. It can be used as an alternative to thrombolysis to restore hemodynamic stability. Martillotti and colleagues[22] reported 3 cases of massive PE during pregnancy or postpartum treated with ECMO and anticoagulation. All women survived, there was no major bleeding, and only 1 premature delivery. Sharma and colleagues[25] described 4 cases of ECMO used during pregnancy (2) and postpartum (2) for respiratory distress. The

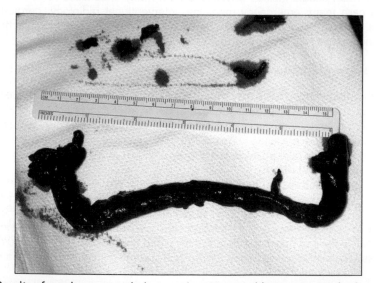

Fig. 3. Results of a pulmonary embolectomy in a 35-year-old woman 1 week after delivery. She was tachycardic and hypotensive in the emergency room and in respiratory distress. Risk factors included her age, hypertension, recent cesarean delivery, and elevated body mass index.

investigators emphasized that pregnancy is not a contraindication to ECMO if there is concern for maternal or fetal survival. If needed, a vaginal or cesarean delivery can be offered to the patient and anticoagulation temporarily held. Intrauterine balloon tamponade can be used if there is postpartum hemorrhage. Survival rates in the series were 80% maternal and 70% fetal. Contraindications to ECMO include severe uncontrollable coagulopathy (disseminated intravascular coagulopathy) or uncontrolled uterine or gastrointestinal hemorrhage.[25]

INFERIOR VENA CAVA FILTERS

The indications for an IVC filter are the same as in nonpregnant patients and include a strong contraindication to anticoagulation, and recurrent VTE events despite adequate anticoagulation and bleeding. There is often a tendency to place an IVC filter antepartum to allow for interruption of anticoagulation around delivery in the patient with a recent acute VTE. According to Fogerty,[10] most women will tolerate temporary interruption of anticoagulation for several hours to permit delivery, and in her opinion there is generally no need for IVC placement during delivery.

Concerns for using an IVC filter include compression from the gravid uterus during pregnancy and an increased risk for lower extremity DVT. In addition, there is a fear for IVC filter thrombosis, perforation, and a failure to retrieve the filter. Others advocate placing a suprarenal IVC filter to decrease the risk of pressure on the IVC filter from the growing uterus. A review of 135 pregnancies using infrarenal or suprarenal filters reported similar complications in both types, suggesting no need for suprarenal IVC filters.[26]

Pregnant women presenting with a submassive or massive PE need to be followed in the intensive care unit. A team of multidisciplinary physicians is needed to manage this critically ill population with expertise in peripartum and postpartum care.[1] Options for the pregnant or postpartum patient in acute PE include thrombolysis, CDT (mechanical or thrombolysis), pulmonary embolectomy, ECMO, or placement of an IVC filter. This team should include physicians from many specialties in addition to the intensive care team: emergency medicine, interventional radiology, cardiothoracic surgeons, vascular surgeons, obstetricians, cardiologists, pharmacologists, hematologists, and vascular medicine physicians.

CANCER AND PULMONARY EMBOLISM

Venous thromboembolism is a major cause of morbidity and mortality in patients with malignancy. It is the second leading cause of death after cancer itself.[27,28] Hospitalization, chemotherapy, and radiation increase the risk of developing VTE in cancer.[28] Additional risk factors are listed in **Box 2**. Patients with cancer are also at a higher risk of bleeding. Intensive care physicians are often charged with managing critically ill patients with cancer and PE.

Overall, there is a threefold to fourfold increased risk of VTE in patients with cancer compared with the general population and up to 20% of all patients with cancer will experience a VTE.[2,31] The incidence of cancer-associated VTE varies depending on the cancer type, time since diagnosis, concurrent treatments, and comorbidities, as listed in **Box 2**. Approximately 25% of patients with malignancy and thrombosis also will require readmission as a result of bleeding or new thrombosis at some point during their treatment.[27]

DIAGNOSIS

The diagnosis of an acute PE in the patient with cancer requires a thorough history, physical examination, and imaging. It may be overlooked because of a nonspecific

---

Box 2
Additional risk factors for venous thromboembolism in patients with cancer

Risk factor(s)
  Age
  Immobilization
  Obesity
  Sedation/mechanical ventilation
  Black race
  Obesity
  Sepsis
  Anemia
  Respiratory or heart failure
  Recent surgery
  Brain tumors
  Lung, pancreatic, and stomach cancers
  Hematologic malignancies (lymphoma)
  Central venous catheterization
  Red blood cell and platelet transfusions

Data from Refs.[29,30]

---

clinical presentation, especially if the patient is in the intensive care unit on a ventilator. The assessment of the patient's pretest probability for a diagnosis of VTE using clinical prediction rules (CPR) followed by the D-dimer has not proven to be as effective as demonstrated in the noncancer population. Peterson and Lee[32] suggest avoiding the CPR and D-dimer in the patient with cancer and proceed directly to imaging. A CUS is generally adequate for the treatment of the hemodynamically stable patient with an acute PE if positive. It may help eliminate the need for CTPA or V/Q scan especially in the critically ill patient not felt stable to transfer for imaging in another area of the hospital. The diagnostic method of choice for acute PE is CTPA.

RISK ASSESSMENT

Risk assessment is recommended to identify patients at highest risk for VTE. The Khorana score has been internally and externally validated and is recommended by the American Society of Clinical Oncology, National Comprehensive Cancer Network, and European Society for Medical Oncology as a tool for predicting chemotherapy-associated VTE using baseline clinical and laboratory variables.[33] Patients at low risk for VTE have 0 points, those with an intermediate risk have 1 to 2 points, and highest risk for VTE ≥3 points. The score is also helpful in educating patients with cancer about the possibility that they may develop thrombosis and identify patients who would benefit from thromboprophylaxis (**Table 2**).

TREATMENT

The treatment of the patient with cancer with an acute submassive or massive PE requiring admission to the intensive care unit may be challenging but should not differ from treatment of the general population, with few exceptions. Treatment options include thrombolysis (systemic or CDT), mechanical thrombectomy, pulmonary embolectomy, or placement of an IVC filter.

Treatment of the patient with cancer is complicated by recurrence of VTE resulting from anticoagulation failure (as high as 10% to 17% treated with warfarin and 6% to

Table 2 The Khorana score	
Patient Characteristic	**Score**
Sites of cancer	
Very high risk (stomach, pancreas)	2
High risk (lung, lymphoma, gynecologic, genitourinary, excluding prostate)	1
Prechemotherapy platelet count $\geq$350,000 mm^3	1
Prechemotherapy leukocyte count >11,000 mm^3	1
Hemoglobin <10 g/dL or use of a erythropoiesis-stimulating agent	1
Body mass index $\geq$35 kg/m^2	1

Data from Khorana AA, Kuderer NM, Culakova E, et al. Development and validation of a predictive model for chemotherapy-associated thrombosis. Blood 2008; 111(10):4902-4907.

9% treated with LMWH) during follow-up.[34] Major or serious bleeding occurs in approximately 7% of patients with cancer-associated thrombosis.[34]

The acute treatment of cancer-associated PE in the critically ill patient is generally initiated with unfractionated heparin (UFH) because of hepatic clearance, an effective antidote, and the ability to monitor its activity. In addition, it is more suitable if there is a need for urgent invasive interventional or surgical procedures given its shorter half-life.

A retrospective cohort study treated 392 patients with acute massive and/or submassive PE (including patients with cancer) used LMWH over UFH with or without thrombolysis.[35] LMWH was favored because of its greater bioavailability, fixed dosing not requiring adjustment, and decreased risk of HIT and concluded it safe and feasible.[35]

The DOACs for patients with cancer are more often used for extended treatment and not in the intensive care unit.[36,37] However, a recent publication by Santos and colleagues[36] used DOACs in intermediate-high risk PE and found them similar in efficacy and safety when compared with LMWH and warfarin.

A common complication that the intensive care physician may see is cancer-associated thrombosis in the setting of thrombocytopenia. The ISTH guidelines recommend patients with a platelet count of $\geq$50 $\times$ 10^9/L receive full-dose anticoagulation without platelet transfusion.[34] If the platelet count is <50 $\times$ 10^9/L, platelet transfusions should be given with full therapeutic anticoagulation to achieve a platelet count >50 $\times$ 10^9/L.[34] If platelet transfusion is not an option, consideration must be given for placement of an IVC filter until the thrombocytopenia resolves.[34]

There are a number of reasons that bleeding occurs in the patient with cancer-associated thrombosis complicating their management. These include chemotherapy-induced thrombocytopenia, metastatic disease, poor nutritional status, impaired renal function, low body weight, decreased mobility, and the need for invasive procedures.[34] The intensive care physician must assess and control the bleeding when it occurs, identify the source, transfuse red blood cells and platelets as needed, and if necessary withhold anticoagulation, unfortunately placing the patient at higher risk for VTE recurrence.

THROMBOLYTIC THERAPY

Thrombolytic therapy for the patient with cancer with a submassive or massive PE may be contraindicated due to underlying thrombocytopenia, a high potential for/or active bleeding, recent surgery, or metastasis to the brain or other vital organs.

A recent retrospective study using the US NIS, Healthcare Cost and Utilization Project Agency for Healthcare Research and Quality database was used to identify hospital admissions for acute PE.[38] The purpose of the study was to determine the association between comorbid cancer and the odds of receiving thrombolysis. This study involved 72,546 admissions for acute PE, of whom 14.7% had comorbid cancer. Thrombolysis was used in only 227 (0.3%) of whom 101 (1.9%) had metastatic disease. In the cancer group, there was a higher odds of in-hospital mortality leading the investigators to conclude that patients with cancer were less likely to receive thrombolytic therapy despite those who presented with hypotension and a clear indication for this treatment.[38]

A study by Casazza and colleagues[39] involving 1702 patients (451 had cancer) also concluded that patients with cancer were less likely to receive thrombolysis compared with patients without cancer. Patients who were clinically unstable at presentation were similar in both cancer and noncancer groups; however, recent surgery was more frequent in the cancer population (18.6% vs 13.7%). Bleeding was the major reason fewer patients with cancer received thrombolysis.[39]

CATHETER-DIRECTED THERAPIES AND PULMONARY EMBOLECTOMY

There are few data regarding CDT and pulmonary embolectomy for acute submassive or massive PE in the patient with cancer. There are several CDT procedures available, including lower-dose thrombolytic therapy using a multi-sidehole infusion catheter with or without the use of ultrasound, and mechanical procedures such as maceration or aspiration thrombectomy. The ESC notes most information on catheter-based embolectomy procedures using mechanical devices or thrombolysis are from registries and case series.[1] Kolkailah and colleagues[40] reviewed their results of 133 patients with submassive PE who underwent surgical pulmonary embolectomy (71) and catheter-directed thrombolysis (62). In their series, 22.6% of the patients had cancer and the indication for advanced treatment was right ventricular strain, recent surgery, or active or recent bleeding. The investigators advocated the use of these 2 advanced treatment options for selected high-risk patients with submassive PE who are not candidates for medical therapy. An analysis from the Society of Thoracic Surgery database included 214 patients of whom most were intermediate-risk PE. In-hospital mortality rates were 12%; however, data on the patient with cancer are not reported.[41] The investigators concluded that surgical pulmonary embolectomy can be performed with acceptable in-hospital outcomes and should be included in the treatment of life-threatening PE.

INFERIOR VENA CAVA FILTERS

Indications for placement of an IVC filter are the same as for the pregnant and postpartum patient listed previously. The risk of recurrence in the patient with cancer not on anticoagulation is particularly high, and insertion of an IVC filter should not delay initiation of anticoagulation once safe to do so.[1]

SUMMARY

Improvements in survival in the patient with cancer may result in more malignancy-related submassive and PEs many of which may be complicated by advanced disease (metastasis or brain involvement), normally a contraindication to thrombolysis. In addition, physicians may be reluctant to perform mechanical thrombectomy or pulmonary embolectomy on this critically ill population, whereas the expertise for these techniques may not be readily available at all hospitals. The patient also may not be stable enough to transfer to another facility for one of these life-saving procedures.[42] This patient population will pose a dilemma in the decision-making process for the intensive care team.

The recent concept of PE response teams (PERTs) has been formed to help navigate the different treatment options for the high-risk patient with PE and will likely help serve the needs for both obstetric patients and patients with cancer. Chaudhury and colleagues[43] analyzed 769 consecutive adult patients admitted with an acute PE diagnosed by CTPA in the 18 months before and after the institution of PERT. The PERT-era patients were found to have lower rates of major or clinically relevant nonmajor bleeding and a significant decrease in 30-day inpatient mortality when compared with the pre-PERT group. The investigators reported that patients with a higher severity of PE seemed to derive the most benefit from the PERT availability.

This concept has gained increasing acceptance by the medical community and is being implemented in hospitals in the United States and worldwide. PERTs bring together a team of specialists from different disciplines to enhance decision-making in the patient with acute submassive and massive PE.[1]

DISCLOSURE

The author have nothing to disclose.

REFERENCES

1. Konstantinides SV, Meyer G, Becattini C, et al. 2019 Guidelines on the diagnosis and management of acute pulmonary embolism. Eur Heart J 2019;40(42):1–61.
2. Konstantinides SV, Torbicki A, Agneilli G, et al. 2014 ESC Guidelines on the diagnosis and management of acute pulmonary embolism. Eur Heart J 2014;35:3033–80.
3. Karon A, Kuklina EV, Hooper CW, et al. Venous thromboembolism as a cause of severe maternal morbidity and mortality in the United States. Semin Perinatol 2019;43:200–4.
4. Jacobsen AF, Skjeldestad FE, Sandset PM. Ante- and postnatal risk factors of venous thrombosis: a hospital –based case control study. J Thromb Haemost 2008;6:905–12.
5. Sultan AA, Tata LJ, West J, et al. Risk factors for first venous thromboembolism around pregnancy: a population-based cohort study from the United Kingdom. Blood 2013;121(19):3953–61.
6. Gammill HS. Postpartum venous thromboembolic risk: one size may not fit all. Blood 2014;124(18):2764–6.
7. James AH, Jamison MG, Brancazio LR, et al. Venous thromboembolism during pregnancy and the postpartum period: incidence, risk factors and mortality. Am J Obstet Gynecol 2006;194(5):1311–5.
8. Ghaji N, Boulet SL, Tepper N, et al. Trends in venous thromboembolism among pregnancy-related hospitalizations, United States, 1994-2009. Am J Obstet Gynecol 2013;209(5):433.e1-8.
9. Macklon NS, Greer IA, Bowman AW. An ultrasound study of gestational and postural changes in the deep venous systems of the leg in pregnancy. Br J Obstet Gynecol 1997;104(2):191–7.
10. Fogerty AE. Management of venous thromboembolism in pregnancy. Curr Treat Options Cardiovasc Med 2018;20:69.

11. Bourjeily G, Paidas M, Khalil H, et al. Pulmonary embolism in pregnancy. Lancet 2010;375(9713):500–12.
12. Kline JA, Richardson DM, Than MP, et al. Systematic review and meta-analysis of pregnant patients investigated for suspected pulmonary embolism in the emergency department. Acad Emerg Med 2014;21:949–59.
13. Righini M, Robert-Ebadi H, Elias A, et al. Diagnosis of pulmonary embolism during pregnancy. A multicenter prospective management outcome study. Ann Intern Med 2018;169:766–73.
14. Dronkers CEA, van der Hulle T, Le Gal G, et al. Towards a tailored diagnostic strategy for future diagnostic studies in pulmonary embolism: communication from the SSC of the ISTH. J Thromb Haemost 2017;15(5):1040–3.
15. van der Pol LM, Tromeur C, Bistervels IM, et al. Pregnancy-adapted YEARS algorithm for diagnosis of suspected pulmonary embolism. N Engl J Med 2019;380: 1139–49.
16. Leung AN, Bull TM, Jaeschke R, et al. An official American Thoracic Society/Society of Thoracic Radiology clinical practice guideline: evaluation of suspected pulmonary embolism in pregnancy. Am J Respir Crit Care Med 2011;184(10): 1200–8.
17. De Carolis S, di Pasquo E, Rossi E, et al. Fondaparinux in pregnancy: could it be a safe option? A review of the literature. Thromb Res 2015;135(6):1049–51.
18. Bernstein SN, Cudemus-Deseda GA, Ortiz VE, et al. Case 33-2019: a 35 year old woman with cardiopulmonary arrest during Cesarean section. N Engl J Med 2019;381:1664–73.
19. Ahearn GS, Hadiliadis D, Govert JA, et al. Massive pulmonary embolism during pregnancy successfully treated with recombinant tissue plasminogen activator: a case report and review of treatment options. Arch Intern Med 2002;162(11): 1221–7.
20. Leonhardt G, Gaul G, Nietsch HH, et al. Thrombolytic therapy in pregnancy. J Thromb Thrombolysis 2006;21(3):271–6.
21. te Raa GD, Ribbert LSM, Snijder RJ, et al. Treatment options in massive pulmonary embolism during pregnancy: a case-report and review of the literature. Thromb Res 2009;124:1–5.
22. Martillotti G, Boehlen F, Robert-Ebadi H, et al. Treatment options for severe pulmonary embolism during pregnancy and the postpartum period: a systematic review. J Thromb Haemost 2017;15:1942–50.
23. Gowda N, Kwabuobi CK, Louis JM. Catheter-directed thrombolytic therapy in the management of massive pulmonary embolism in pregnancy. Obstet Gynecol 2019;134(5):1002–4.
24. Fukuda W, Chiyoya M, Taniguchi S, et al. Management of deep vein thrombosis and pulmonary embolism (venous thromboembolism) during pregnancy. Gen Thorac Cardiovasc Surg 2016;64(6):309–14.
25. Sharma NS, Wille KM, Bellot SC, et al. Modern use of extracorporeal life support in pregnancy and postpartum. ASAIO 2015;61(1):110–4.
26. Harris SA, Velineni R, Davies AH. Inferior vena cava filters in pregnancies: a systemic review. J Vasc Interv Radiol 2016;27(3):354–60.
27. Donnellan E, Khorana AA. Cancer and venous thromboembolic disease: a review. Oncologist 2017;22:199–207.
28. Khorana AA, Francis CW, Culakova E, et al. Thromboembolism is a leading cause of death in cancer patients receiving outpatient chemotherapy. J Thromb Haemost 2007;5:632–4.

29. Khorana AA, Francis CW, Blumberg N, et al. Blood transfusions, thrombosis and mortality in hospitalized patients with cancer. Arch Intern Med 2008;168(21): 2377–81.

30. Heit JA, Silverstein MD, Mohr DN, et al. Risk factors for deep vein thrombosis and pulmonary embolism: a population-based case-control study. Arch Intern Med 2000;160(6):809–15.

31. Sreh A, Nakeshree S, Krishnasamy SK, et al. Therapeutic challenges in the management of acute pulmonary embolism in a cancer patient with chemotherapy-induced thrombocytopenia. Eur J Case Rep Intern Med 2018;5(1):000713.

32. Peterson EA, Lee AYY. Update from the clinic: what's new in the diagnosis of cancer-associated thrombosis? Hematology 2019;1:167–74.

33. Khorana AA, Kuderer NM, Culakova E, et al. Development and validation of a predictive model for chemotherapy-associated thrombosis. Blood 2008;111(10): 4902–7.

34. Carrier M, Khorana AA, Zwicker JI, et al. Management of challenging cases of patients with cancer-associated thrombosis including recurrent thrombosis and bleeding: guidance from the SSC of the ISTH. J Thromb Haemost 2013;11: 1760–5.

35. Ucar EY, Araz O, Akgun M, et al. Low-molecular weight heparin use with thrombolysis: is it effective and safe? Ten years' clinical experience. Respiration 2013; 86:318–23.

36. Santos SM, Cuhna S, Baptista R, et al. Early, real-word experience with direct oral anticoagulants in the treatment of intermediate-high risk acute pulmonary embolism. Rev Port Cardiol 2017;36(11):801–6.

37. Lyman GH, Khorana AA, Kuderer NM, et al. Venous thromboembolism prophylaxis and treatment in patients with cancer: American Society of Clinical Oncology clinical practice guideline update. J Clin Oncol 2013;31(17):2189–204.

38. Weeda ER, Kakamiun KM, Leschorn HX, et al. Comorbid cancer and use of thrombolysis in acute pulmonary embolism. J Thromb Thrombolysis 2019;47: 324–7.

39. Casazza F, Becattini C, Rulli E, et al. Clinical presentation and in-hospital death in acute pulmonary embolism: does cancer matter? Intern Emerg Med 2016;11(6): 817–24.

40. Kolkailah AA, Hirji S, Piazza G, et al. Surgical pulmonary embolectomy and catheter-directed thrombolysis for treatment of submassive pulmonary embolism. J Card Surg 2018;33:252–9.

41. Keeling WB, Sundt T, Leacche M, et al. Outcomes after surgical pulmonary embolectomy for acute pulmonary embolus? A multi-institutional study. Ann Thorac Surg 2016;102:1498–502.

42. Alirezaei T, Hajimoradi B, Pishgahi M, et al. Successfully systemic thrombolytic therapy for massive pulmonary embolism in a patient with breast cancer, brain metastasis and thrombocytopenia: a case report. Clin Case Rep 2018;6:1431–5.

43. Chaudhury P, Gadre S, Schneider E, et al. Impact of multidisciplinary pulmonary embolism response team availability on management and outcomes. Am J Cardiol 2019;124:1465–9.

Post-Intensive Care Unit Follow-up of Pulmonary Embolism

Sonia Jasuja, MD, Richard N. Channick, MD*

KEYWORDS

- Pulmonary embolism • Duration of anticoagulation
- Chronic thromboembolic pulmonary hypertension (CTEPH)
- Post-pulmonary embolism syndrome • Chronic thromboembolic disease (CTED)

KEY POINTS

- The post–intensive care unit follow-up of patients with pulmonary embolism is important to manage anticoagulation and monitor for chronic thromboembolic pulmonary hypertension, chronic thromboembolic disease, or post–pulmonary embolism syndrome.
- The duration of anticoagulation after venous thromboembolism should be determined before hospital discharge and reassessed after 6 months of appropriate anticoagulation.
- Patients should follow-up with a pulmonary vascular disease provider 2 to 12 weeks after acute pulmonary embolism with a follow-up transthoracic echocardiogram.
- We recommend the removal of retrievable inferior vena cava filters as soon as is deemed possible by the patient's pulmonary vascular provider.
- Any patient with persistent dyspnea at more than 12 weeks after the acute event should be evaluated for chronic thromboembolic pulmonary hypertension, chronic thromboembolic disease, or post-pulmonary embolism syndrome.

INTRODUCTION

The post–intensive care unit (ICU) follow-up of patients with intermediate or high-risk pulmonary embolism (PE) is crucial to their comprehensive care. In this article, we discuss the duration of ICU stay, postdischarge follow-up recommendations and intervals, duration of anticoagulation and monitoring for development of post-PE syndrome, chronic thromboembolic disease (CTED) or chronic thromboembolic pulmonary hypertension (CTEPH).

Division of Pulmonary and Critical Care, University of California Los Angeles, David Geffen School of Medicine, 650 Charles East Young Drive South, Room 43-229 CHS, Los Angeles, CA 90095-1690, USA
* Corresponding author.
E-mail address: rchannick@mednet.ucla.edu

Crit Care Clin 36 (2020) 561–570
https://doi.org/10.1016/j.ccc.2020.03.002
0749-0704/20/© 2020 Elsevier Inc. All rights reserved.
criticalcare.theclinics.com

PE is a disease state that leads to significant morbidity and mortality. The 30-day mortality rate for massive PE has been variably reported in different studies, with a range between 12% to as high as 34%.[1,2] The follow-up of these patients is perhaps the most important step in management; the recurrence rate for venous thromboembolism (VTE) events can be as high as 30% and is highest in the time period immediately after the index event.[3] Although the greatest incidence of mortality for patients with massive PE usually occurs during the index hospitalization, the risk of mortality persists after hospitalization for patients with submassive PE.[1] Furthermore, between 0.1% and 9.0% of patients who experience PE go on to develop CTEPH, which can be a life-threatening disease if it is not identified and treated in a timely fashion.[4–11] The Pulmonary Embolism Response Team Consortium Consensus Practice and the 2019 European Society for Cardiology Guidelines for Pulmonary Embolism have published the only consensus guidelines on the follow-up of patients with PE, which we share in this article.[12,13]

DURATION OF INTENSIVE CARE UNIT STAY

The duration of ICU stay varies for patients with PE depending on the severity of presentation and initial risk stratification, as well as their clinical course during the ICU stay. For patients with intermediate risk PE, we recommend at least 24 hours of monitoring in the ICU because of the risk of hemodynamic decompensation to massive PE.[13] In particular, patients who receive catheter-directed therapies or half-dose systemic lysis should be monitored for 24 hours after their advanced therapy is complete. After 24 hours of hemodynamic stability and therapeutic anticoagulation, these intermediate risk patients can be transferred to the general wards before discharge. For patients with hemodynamically significant high-risk PE, we recommend ICU monitoring for the duration of their advanced therapy pending clinical course. Once these high-risk patients are extubated (if applicable), off vasopressor medications, and no longer require any form of life support, we favor monitoring for an additional 24 to 48 hours in the ICU before transfer to the general medical wards. In this group of high-risk patients who have likely received either systemic lysis, catheter-directed lysis or thrombectomy, or surgical embolectomy, we recommend a repeat transthoracic echocardiogram 48 hours after their advanced therapy to assess for improvement in right ventricular (RV) function before transfer out of the ICU.

OUTPATIENT FOLLOW-UP

The primary goal of an outpatient, post-PE follow-up clinic is to monitor for recurrent, persistent or progressive symptoms after PE; determine appropriate plan for type, dosing, duration, and monitoring of anticoagulation; ensure that an appropriate workup is complete regarding underlying factors contributing to the development of the PE, including hypercoagulable workup and age-appropriate cancer screening; facilitate appropriate removal of temporary inferior vena cava (IVC) filters; and last to monitor and identify sequelae of PE, such as post-PE syndrome, CTED, and CTEPH.

The post-PE clinic can be staffed by the members of the Pulmonary Embolism Response Team, such as specialists in pulmonary vascular disease, pulmonary and critical care medicine, cardiology, and/or hematology. We recommend the first visit to the post-PE clinic occur between 2 and 12 weeks after discharge from the hospital.[12,13] The timing of follow-up is based on the patient's clinical course during hospitalization, including the severity of the initial presentation and clinical condition at discharge. For patients with a more tenuous clinical course (eg, patients who required mechanical support, experienced cardiac arrest secondary to their PE, or patients with a high bleeding risk), we recommend clinic follow-up within 2 to 4 weeks of discharge. For other patients with a more stable clinical course, we recommend clinic follow-up 6 to 8 weeks after discharge with a repeat transthoracic echocardiogram scheduled for the same day as the follow-up to evaluate for resolution of RV dysfunction after appropriate therapy.

The first follow-up visit to the post-PE clinic is mainly to discuss plans for anticoagulation; assess for residual, recurrent or progressive symptoms, or residual RV dysfunction after PE; and to complete appropriate hypercoagulable workup and ensure age-appropriate cancer screening is complete. The second follow-up visit to the post-PE clinic should be scheduled 6 months after the index PE event, and the main topics of discussion at this visit are the duration of anticoagulation and assessment for post-PE sequelae, including CTED or CTEPH if the patient remains symptomatic.

Inferior Vena Cava Filter Removal

We recommend expeditious removal of temporary IVC filters as soon as the patient is tolerating therapeutic anticoagulation, which should be within 2 to 4 weeks of IVC filter placement.[13,14] We recommend a multidisciplinary approach to ensure that the IVC filter is removed. First, the procedural team that placed the filter (usually interventional radiology or vascular surgery) should make a 4-week follow-up appointment for outpatient IVC filter removal before the patient's discharge from the hospital. If it is unclear if the filter will be able to be removed by the time of the removal appointment, then the patient should also have a follow-up scheduled in the post-PE clinic within 4 weeks of the PE to assess for the appropriateness of IVC filter removal. If the filter is deemed necessary, then the IVC filter removal should be addressed at regular intervals to ensure that it is not forgotten.

DURATION OF ANTICOAGULATION

The determination of duration of anticoagulation is a critical decision in patients after experiencing PE, because the risk of recurrence is greatest in the months after the PE event and after anticoagulation is stopped.[15] We recommend that all patients with PE receive at least 3 months of therapeutic anticoagulation and at least 6 months of anticoagulation for all patients with PE with a low to moderate bleeding risk.[16] After the initial period of therapeutic anticoagulation is complete, the assessment of recurrence risk of VTE is critical in the decision to stop anticoagulation, continue indefinite therapeutic anticoagulation, or continue extended low-dose anticoagulation.[17]

Recurrence Risk of Venous Thromboembolism

The case-fatality rate for death from recurrent PE is between 4% and 9%, indicating the importance of appropriate dose and duration of anticoagulation after PE.[17] Data from the International Cooperative Pulmonary Embolism Registry demonstrated that 7.9% of patients had recurrent PE within 3 months of their index event, with the mortality of the recurrent PE reaching 33.7% at 14 days after recurrence and 46.8% at 30 days after recurrence.[18] Recurrence rates of VTE are related to the presence or absence of predisposing factors for the development of the initial VTE. As Anderson and Spencer[19] state, the risk factors for the development of VTE are divided into strong, moderate, and weak factors. Strong factors have an odds ratio of greater than 10, whereas moderate factors have an odds ratio of 2 to 9, and weak factors have an odds ratio of less than 2. Furthermore, these factors are divided into patient factors, which generally do not resolve, and environmental factors, which can resolve. In the absence of identifiable predisposing factors for VTE, the recurrence rate in 2 years in 1 study is reported as 20% at 2 years after the initial VTE event.[20] Patients with post-operative VTE have a very low risk of recurrence. Patients with nonsurgical predisposing factors, such as minor surgery, hormone replacement therapy/oral contraceptive pill use, or short hospital admission have a lower recurrence risk of VTE, between 3% and 8% per year. Patients with active malignancy, a history of prior VTE without predisposing factors, or antiphospholipid antibody syndrome have the highest rate of VTE recurrence.[3,13] A study from Denmark by Albertsen and colleagues[21] demonstrated that VTE related to a cancer diagnosis carried the highest recurrence risk. This study looked at recurrence rates for provoked, unprovoked, and cancer-related VTE (including both deep vein thrombosis and PE) at 6 months and 10 years after incident VTE. Recurrence rates at the 6-month follow-up were similar for provoked and unprovoked VTE, whereas results at the 10-year follow-up demonstrated that unprovoked VTE recurrence rates reached those similar to cancer-related VTE recurrence rate.[21]

Anticoagulation in Patients After Pulmonary Embolism Without Cancer

In patients without active malignancy, we recommend all patients be treated with at least 3 to 6 months of therapeutic anticoagulation. Patients in whom this index PE was their first VTE event related to a major transient or reversible predisposing factors, such as major trauma with fractures, surgery under general anesthesia, or fracture of a hip or leg bone, can stop therapeutic anticoagulation after a total of 3 to 6 months from the PE event.[13] In patients with recurrent VTE who have had previous episodes of deep vein thrombosis or PE in whom there are no identifiable predisposing factors, we recommend extended low-dose anticoagulation after 6 months of full-dose anticoagulation is complete with either apixaban 2.5 mg twice daily or rivaroxaban 10 mg daily dosing.[22-25] In patients with antiphospholipid antibody syndrome, we recommend indefinite therapeutic anticoagulation with warfarin with a goal international normalized ratio of 2.5 to 3.5 with a low bleeding risk.[13] In patients with moderate to high bleeding risk and the presence of antiphospholipid antibody syndrome, clinician judgment should be used to determine the appropriate international normalized ratio goal. We also recommend extended low-dose anticoagulation with apixaban or rivaroxaban in patients with a first occurrence of PE and no identifiable risk factors after 6 months of full-dose anticoagulation is complete.[22-25] This strategy should also be considered in patients with a first occurrence of PE in the presence of persistent risk factors, such as inflammatory bowel disease or autoimmune disease, or in patients with minor transient risk factors, such as prolonged travel and oral contraceptive pill or exogenous hormone use.[13]

During our second post-PE clinic visit at 6 months after the VTE event, we obtain repeat lower extremity venous duplex ultrasounds in patients who presented with deep vein thrombosis in addition to their index PE event. If these patients have evidence of residual deep vein thrombosis or progression of deep vein thrombosis from previous examinations, we recommend keeping these patients on full-dose anticoagulation, as opposed to extended low-dose anticoagulation or stopping anticoagulation given the increased risk of recurrence with residual deep vein thrombosis.[26]

Bleeding Risk

There are several bleeding risk calculators that can be used when assessing bleeding risk among this patient population. The HAS-BLED, ATRIA, and

HEMORR2HAGES scores are all used in atrial fibrillation but can be applied in the setting of VTE as well.[27–29] Furthermore, for VTE-related bleeding risk, the RIETE score was developed specifically for VTE patients.[30] In patients with a high risk of bleeding with an indication for lifelong, indefinite, full-dose or extended dose anticoagulation, we do not stop anticoagulation. If these patients experience a serious bleeding event requiring hospitalization, anticoagulation can be preferably switched to continuous intravenous unfractionated heparin with a lower partial thromboplastin time goal or stopped. In the event of life-threatening bleeding, such as intracranial bleed or hemorrhagic shock, an IVC filter should be placed and the appropriate anticoagulation reversal agent should be used. Anticoagulation should be resumed as soon as possible, preferably under direct monitoring while the patient is still hospitalized to ensure that the source of the bleeding has been treated adequately without a repeat bleed. In cases of patients who are of advanced age (>75 years) or in patients with advanced-stage comorbid illness, we stop anticoagulation after a bleeding event.

In patients with a low to moderate risk of bleeding, we do not alter our recommendations for anticoagulation, as discussed elsewhere in this article.

Recurrent Venous Thromboembolism Prediction Tools

In patients with a first episode of PE without predisposing factors, we use the Vienna prediction model to calculate the 1- and 5-year risks of recurrent VTE events. We use this tool as an adjunct during our discussions with patients in our shared decision making discussions regarding the duration of anticoagulation.[31,32] Another tool is the DASH prediction score, which uses similar factors to determine recurrence risk of VTE in patients who have experienced unprovoked VTE.[33]

Anticoagulation in Patients After Pulmonary Embolism with Cancer

Patients with active malignancy should receive therapeutic anticoagulation indefinitely after their first VTE event in the setting of active malignancy, given the high risk of recurrence of VTE in the setting of active malignancy.[21,34]

ASSESSMENT FOR POST–PULMONARY EMBOLISM SEQUELAE, INCLUDING CHRONIC THROMBOEMBOLIC PULMONARY HYPERTENSION, CHRONIC THROMBOEMBOLIC DISEASE, AND POST–PULMONARY EMBOLISM SYNDROME

Acute PE may progress to chronic PE and CTED/CTEPH in 1% to 4% of patients.[4,5,35,36] Patients who present to the post-PE clinic with persistent or progressive pulmonary symptoms, including dyspnea at rest or exertion, presyncope or syncope, chest pain, or exercise intolerance, should be evaluated further. Post-PE syndrome can range from mild deconditioning to severe pulmonary hypertension, that is, CTEPH.[37] CTEPH should be considered in patients with persistent pulmonary symptoms after 3 months of anticoagulation who have at least 1 persistent lobar or segmental unmatched perfusion defect on ventilation/perfusion (V/Q) imaging and evidence of pulmonary hypertension on right heart catheterization, defined as mean pulmonary artery pressure of more than 20 mm Hg, a pulmonary capillary wedge pressure of less than 15 mm Hg, and a pulmonary vascular resistance of greater than 3 woods units.[38,39] CTED is diagnosed in patients with pulmonary symptoms after 3 months of anticoagulation who have at least 1 persistent lobar or segmental unmatched perfusion defect on V/Q imaging without evidence of pulmonary hypertension on right heart catheterization at rest.[37,39] Although there are no defined diagnostic criteria, post-PE syndrome is diagnosed in patients with persistent dyspnea and exercise intolerance who may or may not have residual evidence of perfusion defect on V/Q scan with documented exercise limitation on cardiopulmonary exercise testing as evidenced by a percent predicted Vo_2 peak of less than 80%.[37,40]

Although the incidence of CTEPH after PE is relatively low, the detection of CTEPH is of paramount importance to the well-being of these patients because CTEPH is a severe, progressive, and life-threatening disease process that has a cure if identified appropriately.[10,41] The cure for CTEPH is pulmonary endarterectomy; however, 20% to 40% of patients are not surgical candidates at the time of diagnosis.[35,36,42,43] In these nonsurgical patients, possible treatment options include balloon pulmonary angioplasty or medical therapy depending on the clinical characteristics of each patient.[39,44-49]

Prevalence of Chronic Thromboembolic Pulmonary Hypertension and Post–Pulmonary Embolism Syndrome After Pulmonary Embolism

The prevalence of CTEPH after PE ranges between 0.1% and 9.1%, depending on which study is used.[4-11] This large range in prevalence can be elucidated by differences in study design, including screening protocols and inclusion criteria. Klok and colleagues[50] evaluated all patients diagnosed with PE by screening echocardiography. Patients with echocardiographic evidence of pulmonary hypertension underwent complete workup for CTEPH evaluation, and the incidence of CTEPH in this study was 0.57%. In a study by Hsu and colleagues,[4] 4% of patients with acute PE were diagnosed with CTEPH, with a median time from PE event to CTEPH development of 36 months. This study goes further to demonstrate that echocardiographic measures of RV function, as opposed to echocardiographic estimates of pulmonary artery pressure, are more predictive of development of CTEPH.[4] Studies that used only echocardiography to diagnose CTEPH without confirmatory right heart catheterization testing found a higher prevalence of CTEPH compared with studies that diagnosed CTEPH by right heart catheterization, angiography, and/or V/Q scintigraphy.[5-11,50] Furthermore, the ELOPE cohort study demonstrated that 46.5% of patients have a persistent percent-predicted Vo_2 of less than 80% at 1 year after a PE event.[51]

Risk Factors for the Development of Chronic Thromboembolic Pulmonary Hypertension

There have been several studies conducted to evaluate possible risk factors for the development of CTEPH. Klok and colleagues[52] followed patients after acute PE and identified 6 factors that were independently associated with the diagnosis of CTEPH: unprovoked PE, known hypothyroidism, symptom onset more than 2 weeks before the diagnosis of PE, the presence of RV dysfunction on computed tomography scans or echocardiography, a known history of diabetes mellitus, and thrombolytic therapy or embolectomy. Another study from France demonstrated that older age, multiple previous VTE events, proximal PE, higher levels of brain natriuretic peptide and higher systolic pulmonary artery pressures were associated with the presence of CTEPH after a PE event.[5] Furthermore, Bonderman and colleagues[42,53] discuss that certain medical conditions, such as splenectomy, ventriculoatrial shunt, inflammatory bowel disease, and osteomyelitis, are risk factors for the development of CTEPH and the presence of these associated medical conditions actually predict increased operative risk and worse long-term outcomes in patients with CTEPH undergoing pulmonary endarterectomy.[54]

Workup of Chronic Thromboembolic Pulmonary Hypertension, Chronic Thromboembolic Disease, and Post–Pulmonary Embolism Syndrome

During the 6-month follow-up visit in the post-PE clinic, we evaluate patients for symptoms of persistent or recurrent dyspnea and exercise intolerance. If these symptoms are present, we recommend obtaining a repeat transthoracic echocardiogram and a V/Q scintigraphy scan to further evaluate for possible CTEPH, CTED, or post-PE syndrome.[12,13] A normal V/Q scintigraphy scan without the presence of unmatched perfusion defects is a highly sensitive test for ruling out CTEPH. If the V/Q scintigraphy scan is abnormal and concerning for CTEPH, we refer the patient for evaluation in our CTEPH center, with a plan for a pulmonary angiogram and discussion of the patient's case in our multidisciplinary CTEPH conference to determine next best treatment plan.[12,13,39]

SUMMARY

The follow-up of patients in a dedicated post-PE clinic or by a Pulmonary Embolism Response Team is of utmost importance in the prevention of recurrent VTE events. Regular follow-up after PE allows for assessment of RV function, determination of an appropriate anticoagulation dose and duration and monitoring for post-PE sequelae, including CTEPH, CTED, and post-PE syndrome.

DISCLOSURE

The authors have nothing to disclose.

REFERENCES

1. Secemsky E, Chang Y, Jain CC, et al. Contemporary management and outcomes of patients with massive and submassive pulmonary embolism. Am J Med 2018; 131(12):1506–14.e0.
2. Jimenez D, de Miguel-Díez J, Guijarro R, et al. Trends in the management and outcomes of acute pulmonary embolism: analysis from the RIETE registry. J Am Coll Cardiol 2016;67(2):162–70.
3. Heit JA. The epidemiology of venous thromboembolism in the community. Arterioscler Thromb Vasc Biol 2008;28(3):370–2.
4. Hsu C-H, Lin C-C, Li W-T, et al. Right ventricular dysfunction is associated with the development of chronic thromboembolic pulmonary hypertension but not with mortality post-acute pulmonary embolism. Medicine (Baltimore) 2019; 98(48):e17953.
5. Guerin L, Couturaud F, Parent F, et al. Prevalence of chronic thromboembolic pulmonary hypertension after acute pulmonary embolism. Prevalence of CTEPH after pulmonary embolism. Thromb Haemost 2014;112(3):598–605.
6. Becattini C, Agnelli G, Pesavento R, et al. Incidence of chronic thromboembolic pulmonary hypertension after a first episode of pulmonary embolism. Chest 2006; 130(1):172–5.
7. Dentali F, Donadini M, Gianni M, et al. Incidence of chronic pulmonary hypertension in patients with previous pulmonary embolism. Thromb Res 2009;124(3): 256–8.
8. Miniati M, Monti S, Bottai M, et al. Survival and restoration of pulmonary perfusion in a long-term follow-up of patients after acute pulmonary embolism. Medicine (Baltimore) 2006;85(5):253–62.

9. Poli D, Grifoni E, Antonucci E, et al. Incidence of recurrent venous thromboembolism and of chronic thromboembolic pulmonary hypertension in patients after a first episode of pulmonary embolism. J Thromb Thrombolysis 2010;30(3):294–9.

10. Surie S, Gibson NS, Gerdes VEA, et al. Active search for chronic thromboembolic pulmonary hypertension does not appear indicated after acute pulmonary embolism. Thromb Res 2010;125(5):e202–5.

11. Park JS, Ahn J, Choi JH, et al. The predictive value of echocardiography for chronic thromboembolic pulmonary hypertension after acute pulmonary embolism in Korea. Korean J Intern Med 2017;32(1):85–94.

12. Rivera-Lebron B, McDaniel M, Ahrar K, et al. Diagnosis, treatment and follow up of acute pulmonary embolism: consensus Practice from the PERT Consortium. Clin Appl Thromb Hemost 2019;25. 1076029619853037.

13. Konstantinides SV, Meyer G, Becattini C, et al. 2019 ESC guidelines for the diagnosis and management of acute pulmonary embolism developed in collaboration with the European Respiratory Society (ERS): the Task Force for the diagnosis and management of acute pulmonary embolism of the European Society of Cardiology (ESC). Eur Heart J 2020;41(4):543–603.

14. Members ATF, Torbicki A, Perrier A, et al. Guidelines on the diagnosis and management of acute pulmonary embolism: the task force for the diagnosis and management of acute pulmonary embolism of the European Society of Cardiology (ESC). Eur Heart J 2008;29(18):2276–315.

15. Boutitie F, Pinede L, Schulman S, et al. Influence of preceding length of anticoagulant treatment and initial presentation of venous thromboembolism on risk of recurrence after stopping treatment: analysis of individual participants' data from seven trials. BMJ 2011;342:d3036.

16. Kearon C, Akl EA, Ornelas J, et al. Antithrombotic therapy for VTE disease. Chest 2016;149(2):315–52.

17. Douketis JD, Gu CS, Schulman S, et al. The risk for fatal pulmonary embolism after discontinuing anticoagulant therapy for venous thromboembolism. Ann Intern Med 2007;147(11):766–74.

18. Goldhaber SZ, Visani L, De Rosa M. Acute pulmonary embolism: clinical outcomes in the International Cooperative Pulmonary Embolism Registry (ICOPER). Lancet 1999;353(9162):1386–9.

19. Anderson FAJ, Spencer FA. Risk factors for venous thromboembolism. Circulation 2003;107(23 Suppl 1):I9–16.

20. Baglin T, Luddington R, Brown K, et al. Incidence of recurrent venous thromboembolism in relation to clinical and thrombophilic risk factors: prospective cohort study. Lancet 2003;362(9383):523–6.

21. Albertsen IE, Nielsen PB, Sogaard M, et al. Risk of recurrent venous thromboembolism: a Danish Nationwide cohort study. Am J Med 2018;131(9):1067–74.e4.

22. Agnelli G, Buller HR, Cohen A, et al. Apixaban for extended treatment of venous thromboembolism. N Engl J Med 2013;368(8):699–708.

23. Agnelli G, Buller HR, Cohen A, et al. Oral apixaban for the treatment of acute venous thromboembolism. N Engl J Med 2013;369(9):799–808.

24. Bauersachs R, Berkowitz SD, Brenner B, et al. Oral rivaroxaban for symptomatic venous thromboembolism. N Engl J Med 2010;363(26):2499–510.

25. Buller HR, Prins MH, Lensin AWA, et al. Oral rivaroxaban for the treatment of symptomatic pulmonary embolism. N Engl J Med 2012;366(14):1287–97.

26. Siragusa S, Malato A, Anastasio R, et al. Residual vein thrombosis to establish duration of anticoagulation after a first episode of deep vein thrombosis: the

Duration of Anticoagulation based on Compression UltraSonography (DACUS) study. Blood 2008;112(3):511–5.

27. Lip GYH, Frison L, Halperin JL, et al. Comparative validation of a novel risk score for predicting bleeding risk in anticoagulated patients with atrial fibrillation: the HAS-BLED (hypertension, abnormal renal/liver function, stroke, bleeding history or predisposition, labile INR, elderly, drugs/alcohol concomitantly) score. J Am Coll Cardiol 2011;57(2):173–80.

28. Fang MC, Go AS, Chang Y, et al. A new risk scheme to predict warfarin-associated hemorrhage: the ATRIA (Anticoagulation and Risk Factors in Atrial Fibrillation) Study. J Am Coll Cardiol 2011;58(4):395–401.

29. Gage BF, Yan Y, Milligan PE, et al. Clinical classification schemes for predicting hemorrhage: results from the National Registry of Atrial Fibrillation (NRAF). Am Heart J 2006;151(3):713–9.

30. Nieto JA, Solano R, Ruiz-Ribo MD, et al. Fatal bleeding in patients receiving anti-coagulant therapy for venous thromboembolism: findings from the RIETE registry. J Thromb Haemost 2010;8(6):1216–22.

31. Eichinger S, Heinze G, Jandeck LM, et al. Risk assessment of recurrence in patients with unprovoked deep vein thrombosis or pulmonary embolism: the Vienna prediction model. Circulation 2010;121(14):1630–6.

32. Marcucci M, Iorio A, Douketis JD, et al. Risk of recurrence after a first unprovoked venous thromboembolism: external validation of the Vienna Prediction Model with pooled individual patient data. J Thromb Haemost 2015;13(5):775–81.

33. Tosetto A, Iorio A, Marcucci M, et al. Predicting disease recurrence in patients with previous unprovoked venous thromboembolism: a proposed prediction score (DASH). J Thromb Haemost 2012;10(6):1019–25.

34. Exter den PL, Kooiman J, Huisman MV. Validation of the Ottawa prognostic score for the prediction of recurrent venous thromboembolism in patients with cancer-associated thrombosis. J Thromb Haemost 2013;11(5):998–1000.

35. Pepke-Zaba J, Delcroix M, Lang I, et al. Chronic thromboembolic pulmonary hypertension (CTEPH). Circulation 2011;124(18):1973–81.

36. Kim NH, Lang IM. Risk factors for chronic thromboembolic pulmonary hypertension. Eur Respir Rev 2012;21(123):27–31.

37. Sista AK, Klok FA. Late outcomes of pulmonary embolism: the post-PE syndrome. Thromb Res 2018;164:157–62.

38. Simonneau G, Montani D, Celermajer DS, et al. Haemodynamic definitions and updated clinical classification of pulmonary hypertension. Eur Respir J 2019; 53(1):1801913.

39. Kim NH, Delcroix M, Jaïs X, et al. Chronic thromboembolic pulmonary hypertension. Eur Respir J 2019;53(1):1801915.

40. Klok FA, van der Hulle T, Exter den PL, et al. The post-PE syndrome: a new concept for chronic complications of pulmonary embolism. Blood Rev 2014; 28(6):221–6.

41. Jamieson SW. Historical perspective: surgery for chronic thromboembolic disease. Semin Thorac Cardiovasc Surg 2006;18(3):218–22.

42. Bonderman D, Skoro-Sajer N, Jakowitsch J, et al. Predictors of outcome in chronic thromboembolic pulmonary hypertension. Circulation 2007;115(16): 2153–8.

43. Mayer E. Surgical and post-operative treatment of chronic thromboembolic pulmonary hypertension. Eur Respir Rev 2010;19(115):64.

44. Ghofrani H-A, D'Armini AM, Grimminger F, et al. Riociguat for the treatment of chronic thromboembolic pulmonary hypertension. N Engl J Med 2013;369(4): 319–29.
45. Ghofrani H-A, Galie N, Grimminger F, et al. Riociguat for the treatment of pulmonary arterial hypertension. N Engl J Med 2013;369(4):330–40.
46. Simonneau G, D'Armini AM, Ghofrani H-A, et al. Riociguat for the treatment of chronic thromboembolic pulmonary hypertension: a long-term extension study (CHEST-2). Eur Respir J 2015;45(5):1293–302.
47. Ghofrani H-A, Simonneau G, D'Armini AM, et al. Macitentan for the treatment of inoperable chronic thromboembolic pulmonary hypertension (MERIT-1): results from the multicentre, phase 2, randomised, double-blind, placebo-controlled study. Lancet Respir Med 2017;5(10):785–94.
48. Mizoguchi H, Ogawa A, Munemasa M, et al. Refined balloon pulmonary angioplasty for inoperable patients with chronic thromboembolic pulmonary hypertension. Circ Cardiovasc Interv 2012;5(6):748–55.
49. Sugimura K, Fukumoto Y, Satoh K, et al. Percutaneous transluminal pulmonary angioplasty markedly improves pulmonary hemodynamics and long-term prognosis in patients with chronic thromboembolic pulmonary hypertension. Circ J 2012;76(2):485–8.
50. Klok FA, van Kralingen KW, van Dijk APJ, et al. Prospective cardiopulmonary screening program to detect chronic thromboembolic pulmonary hypertension in patients after acute pulmonary embolism. Haematologica 2010;95(6):970.
51. Kahn SR, Akaberi A, Granton JT, et al. Quality of life, dyspnea, and functional exercise capacity following a first episode of pulmonary embolism: results of the ELOPE cohort study. Am J Med 2017;130(8):990.e9-21.
52. Klok FA, Dzikowska-Diduch O, Kostrubiec M, et al. Derivation of a clinical prediction score for chronic thromboembolic pulmonary hypertension after acute pulmonary embolism. J Thromb Haemost 2015;14(1):121–8.
53. Bonderman D, Jakowitsch J, Adlbrecht C, et al. Medical conditions increasing the risk of chronic thromboembolic pulmonary hypertension. Thromb Haemost 2005;93(3):512–6.
54. Jaïs X, Ioos V, Jardim C, et al. Splenectomy and chronic thromboembolic pulmonary hypertension. Thorax 2005;60(12):1031.

Moving?

Make sure your subscription moves with you!

To notify us of your new address, find your **Clinics Account Number** (located on your mailing label above your name), and contact customer service at:

Email: journalscustomerservice-usa@elsevier.com

800-654-2452 (subscribers in the U.S. & Canada)
314-447-8871 (subscribers outside of the U.S. & Canada)

Fax number: 314-447-8029

Elsevier Health Sciences Division
Subscription Customer Service
3251 Riverport Lane
Maryland Heights, MO 63043

*To ensure uninterrupted delivery of your subscription, please notify us at least 4 weeks in advance of move.

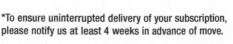

Printed and bound by CPI Group (UK) Ltd, Croydon, CR0 4YY

03/10/2024

01040479-0013